Crossfit

How To Lose Weight With Crossfit Routines And Exercises

(Learn More About Crossfit Training Reaching Your Fitness Goals)

Raymond Baker

Published By **Elena Holly**

Raymond Baker

All Rights Reserved

*Crossfit: How To Lose Weight With Crossfit
Routines And Exercises (Learn More About Crossfit
Training Reaching Your Fitness Goals)*

ISBN 978-1-77485-560-7

No part of this guidebook shall be reproduced in any form without permission in writing from the publisher except in the case of brief quotations embodied in critical articles or reviews.

Legal & Disclaimer

The information contained in this ebook is not designed to replace or take the place of any form of medicine or professional medical advice. The information in this ebook has been provided for educational & entertainment purposes only.

The information contained in this book has been compiled from sources deemed reliable, and it is accurate to the best of the Author's knowledge; however, the Author cannot guarantee its accuracy and validity and cannot be held liable for any errors or omissions. Changes are periodically made to this book. You must consult your doctor or get professional medical advice before using any of the suggested remedies, techniques, or information in this book.

Upon using the information contained in this book, you agree to hold harmless the Author from and against any damages, costs, and expenses, including any legal fees potentially resulting from the application of any of the information provided by this guide. This disclaimer applies to any damages or injury caused by the use and application, whether directly or indirectly, of any advice or information presented, whether for breach of contract, tort, negligence, personal injury, criminal intent, or under any other cause of action.

You agree to accept all risks of using the information presented inside this book. You need to consult a professional medical practitioner in order to ensure you are both able and healthy enough to participate in this program.

Table of contents

Introduction

In this day and age, we all know that making fitness a part of your life should be a high priority in everyone's life -- it should become a daily habit, the same as brushing your teeth or taking a shower. Dedicating a little bit of time each day isn't much to ask when you take into account all the positive things you achieve just by being physically fit. Apart from looking and feeling great, working out can benefit you in the following areas as well:

* Help reduce blood pressure
* Increase flexibility, which can help prevent injury and help with muscular tension.
* Help to relieve stress, depression and anxiety
* Help with gaining muscle, which can build and maintain strong bones
* Keep your heart healthy and reduce the risk of heart disease
* Lower the risk of developing colon cancer
* Increase your ability to concentrate, think

faster   and   become   more   sharp And remember it isn't necessary for you to be in a gym to be fit. What you are about to discover shortly will show you many exercises that can be performed outdoors, at home and anywhere else you like. That's the beauty of CrossFit training!

You can enjoy fitness with your kids, your spouse, family or friends, people of all ages can participate.

CrossFit training is taking the world by storm and is reported to be growing by 350% each year which appears to be accurate with more and more exposure since the CrossFit games are shown all over the world through ESPN and is fast becoming the elite competition for fitness bragging rights. So through this guide you will discover the history of CrossFit training, the benfits of CrossFit, the best exercises that will get you at your peak fitness levels and a whole lot more. So before we do that, to start off we must go to the beginning...

Chapter 1: What Is Crossfit Training

Many of sports enthusiasts are becoming interested in CrossFit training nowadays. Actually, this training combines a lot of effective routines that enable one to create diversity in workout.

On the other hand, sports medicine experts consider this training as a balanced and holistic way of attaining fitness and health in just a short period of time. Like when gaining stamina, choose either to do swimming, biking and basketball several days in a week.

In doing so, a person is allowed to enjoy a variety of training which can be fun and exciting while getting the desired fitness goals.

Dating back in history, CrossFit Training was started by Greg Class, a high school gymnast who was along with his wife named Lauren Glassman. CrossFit became associated with the first gymnasium in 1995. In that same year, Santa Cruz police department hired Lauren Glassman to be able to train the troops. For seven consecutive weeks, the "Gagetown Infantry School" was focused in various tests in fitness categories that include strength, agility, stamina, flexibility, balance, accuracy, speed, power, coordination and respiratory endurance. With the many categories, CrossFit also scored the highest.

As a result, gym trainers became satisfied because of the workout results. Gymnasiums that are affiliated with CrossFit have grown swiftly. In 2005, there were only eighteen that rose to one thousand seven hundred gymnasiums in 2010. Weightlifting coaches like Louie Simmons, Mike Burgener and Bill Starr partnered with the CrossFit organization.

Cross Fit is a health program that is greatly designed to optimize and bring the body to it's peak performance levels. Nevertheless, the nature of this training program is not involved with any of the risks. So far, the benefits of CrossFit training far outweigh the risks. When done in limited time and in poor form, different CrossFit exercises might elevate the risk of injury if performed incorrectly. So, This should

4

not be performed by people without getting proper supervision first.

CrossFit And Its Effect On The Body- All of the parts of the human body are conditioned for them to function well. Through the exercise variations within CrossFit training, the body is allowed to develop various muscle groups. The focus is not only on a single group of muscles, but on all the body muscles as well. Shifting from a single activity to the next makes you exercise the various muscles group for a balanced training.

Crossfit exercises may likely prevent boredom. One of the common problems in doing an exercise regimen is when you become bored. You suddenly become not interested in it that you usually end up quitting. Remember that in CrossFit training, one can choose from a wide range of exercises each day, thus making the training more interesting. With varied routines, you can look forward to a variety of workouts.

Crossfit training has no fixed schedule, which makes it flexible. If circumstances have gone beyond your control, it may likely prevent you from the regular morning runs in the city park. There are still productive trainings that can be done like swimming in the morning or playing lawn tennis at night. The good thing about it is that you can adjust your training around anything you like.

So now that you have learnt a bit about what CrossFit training is, it's time we covered the history of this fitness phenomenon

Chapter 2: The History Of Crossfit Training

Cross fit training is a form of physical training which is intended to develop your power and your strength. This is a form of training which became popular in the year 2000. Because of the undeniable nature of CrossFit exercises, there are lots of people who have been addicted to it. In fact, this form of training is already gaining popularity these days. There are so many people from the different parts of the world who are eager to learn this training. Though the overall nature of CrossFit training might be highly challenging enough, this routine is worth performing. If you are one of those people who are looking forward to learning this form of training, it is now important for you to know a little bit of its history.

The actual founder of CrossFit training is Greg Glassman. He was a professional gymnast during his time. Though the training has boomed in the year 2000, it started being offered by gyms in the year 1995. The training itself focuses in terms of conditioning your body. This comes with different methodologies which are intended in order to provide general and broad physical fitness through the myriad of exercises you can perform. Examples of the activities under Greg Glassman are gymnastics, sprinting, weightlifting and others. These were basically the first exercises introduced under this kind of exercise. However, new components of the training have already been added. These have made the training more intense and challenging.

Specifically, the first gym that has offered CrossFit training is CrossFit North, which is locafed in Seattle, Washington. The coaches who have contributed a lot in the development of CrossFit training are Mike Burgener, Bob Harpe and Louie Simmons. In addition to that, there was a great help from Dr. Nicholas Romanov who is a subject matter expert, that led to the success of the training. Romanov is the inventor of Pose Method of running. In the recent years, several variations have also been included in the training. Among the individuals who are responsible for these changes are Robb Wolf, Mark Rippetoe and Mark Twight.

Since the introduction of this form of training, so many people have experienced major benefits of CrossFit training. Usually, people who undergo this form of training will experience enhanced balanced, agility, speed, flexibility, power and endurance. As of now, the popularity of this training is still at its height. In the year 2005, there were a total of 15 gyms and fitness institutions offering this kind of training. In the span of a half decade, the popularity of the training even increased. Based from the information released in the year 2010, there were 1,700 fitness institutions and gyms offering this form of training. It is also expected that the number of fitness institutions offering CrossFit training will continue to increase these days. As of now, it is expected that the numbers of fitness institutions and gyms offering CrossFit training will increased tremendously for up to 3,400.

Way back in the year 1970, Greg Glassman did not have any clue that this training will be used after 3 decades. According to one of his interviews, he primarily developed this concept just for the sake of his colleagues and of course, himself. He never thought that some fitness enthusiasts from the other parts of the world will embrace the benefits of CrossFit training.

Most of those individuals who tried this kind of training are highly satisfied with its results because it brought out the best in them. For this reason, there are even greater numbers of fitness instructors who are studying the CrossFit training. Examples of these coaches who have devoted some of their time in learning CrossFit training are Mike Burgener, Louie Simmons and Bill Starr who have trained together with John Welbourn. Once you finish this program, you will receive certification seminars concerning running and endurance, kettle bells, gymnastics weightlifting and others. If you want to learn this program, it is important that you apply in a legitimate instructor so that you will be given the right training methods.

These are some of the things you need to keep in mind when it comes to the history of CrossFit training. Surely, it pays a lot to know a little background of this form of training before you actually do it. Unlike the other kinds of trainings, Greg Glassman never thought that the world will appreciate this form of exercise than what he has imagined. Over the years, expect that there will also be additional enhancements in this form of training. For sure, these enhancements will make CrossFit training a lot better than before. So, why don't you perform it now? You will surely achieve the body you have always dreamed of.

Chapter 3: Benefits Of Crossfit Training

It is very impressive that there are more and more people who are becoming health-conscious. In fact, there are many men and women from all over the world looking for the edge when it comes to fitness. So this is where CrossFit training comes into play, Since this is a very effective way of molding your body and gaining tremendous fitness. So now let's discover the benefits of CrossFit training

One of the benefits of CrossFit training is that it comes with efficient and fast results. Usually, you only have to exert some time in doing CrossFit training. Expect that at the end of the training, you will notice that your muscle has developed a greater strength and that your overall fitness level has improved. You will also notice that your power has become better as compared to those people who make use of the traditional workouts in fitness institutions. However, you have to make sure that you perform the workout properly to experience its optimal effects in just a short period of time.

In addition to the list of benefits of CrossFit training, this is also a well-rounded kind of routine. When exercising, it is important to ensure that your whole body is involved. This is to ensure that you have a proportioned and well-toned body unlike those who only focus in a specific part of their body. Since CrossFit training makes use of a holistic approach, expect that there are different workout styles that will make your entire body fitter.

Most of the time, fitness enthusiasts tend to cheat and give up in performing their routines because they feel bored with their routine. In the case of CrossFit exercises, you will not feel bored. In every single day, you can choose from a variety of workouts called WOD (Work Out of the Day). In fact, you will never get bored and you might find yourself increasingly becoming interested in your workouts day by day.

Another nice benefit of CrossFit training is that this is affordable. In terms of performing the exercises you need to do, there is no need for you to secure different equipment in the future. Most of the components of the workout set your body in motion in order to achieve a fitter physique. This is far different from the other kinds of routines wherein you are obliged to purchase your own equipment for your exercises to be performed efficiently. Surely, this is one of the benefits that you will like the most about this program.

In addition to the benefits of CrossFit training mentioned, this form of training is also effective in terms of conditioning your own body before undergoing any kind of routine. This makes your body unable to feel any stress. Before you are introduced to a new routine, your trainers will first prepare your system through the introduction of some preparatory exercise routines. As you do the complex routines in the future, you will not experience too much difficulty. This is far different as compared to the other kinds of exercise routines offered in some fitness institutions.

These are some of the benefits that you can get in performing CrossFit training. This is indeed one of the most promising routines that you can try to give you the kind of body you have always wanted to have. It is important that if you want to experience the benefits of CrossFit training, you should only trust undergo trained experts or instructors who will handle such training. This is because of the fact that the training is a specialized form of exercise. Without proper skills and knowledge about the program, it is impossible for you to experience the benefits of CrossFit training. So, now let's turn to the different exercises of CrossFit!

Chapter 4: Crossfit Exercises

Cross fit training is considered as a series of exercises that is intended to improve your conditioning and strength. Basically, CrossFit training focuses primarily in weightlifting under the Olympic style. There are different routines that you can do when you are planning to try this form of training. Mostly, the exercises are able to exercise most of your body parts. Because of the holistic approach of this training, it would be easier for you to achieve the body that you have always wanted to have. If you do undergo this form of training, it is important for you to know some of the CrossFit exercises that you might do in the future.

Cindy Routine is one of the CrossFit exercises that can tone your body. Basically, this is a form of full body exercise and strategy, which include pushups as well as body weight squats. Cindy Routine comes with a time frame of about 20 minutes. This should be performed the next day, and the athlete should make sure that progress is there. Though this routine can be performed very quickly, this is one of the best fat burning routines under CrossFit exercises. In addition to that, Cindy Routine is also designed in order to add extra mass of muscles in your chest and in your shoulders. Thus, this gives you weight loss and body sculpturing effects.

Filthy 50 is also considered as one of the best CrossFit exercises. Unlike the first one, this is a very demanding and rigorous kind of workout. This requires you to do 50 repetitions of 10 varieties of exercises such as double unders, burpee, ball shots, back extension, push press, lifts, lunge steps, kettleball swings, pull-ups and box jumps. Even if this kind of routine is highly demanding, it will still offer your body with the fastest means to lose weight and to burn extra calories even in one session only. That is why weight loss is definitely one of the benefits of CrossFit training particularly in performing this routine.

Cross fit training is also composed of the exercise called Thrusters and Pull Ups. This is also a workout that should be done in a repetitive manner. You can begin the routine by performing as many push-ups and thrusters as you can. Once you feel that you are already exhausted and you have already done all the maximum repetitions, you can slow down. This is an exercise that is efficient in burning the calories and excess fats present in your stomach area.

L-sit is also included in the CrossFit exercises that you can perform in the future. Because of the nature of this exercise, it is best for your stomach and for your abs. Usually, you can lose portion of your excess fat in stomach in performing this routine. Under this exercise, your body is being supported by your arms while your legs are straight on your front.

Double Under is also another addition to your CrossFit exercises. This is basically a form of jump rope exercise that will increase the rush of your adrenaline. This is being performed by simply jumping over the rope, ensuring that the rope will pass two times before you land on the floor. This routine will require you to have increased work capacity. In turn, this will enhance the calorie burning effects of the exercise. Thus, this will give you the chance to lose weight easily.

Dead Lift Plus Run is also another component of CrossFit training. The combination of running and dead lift makes this routine considered as a potent one. This will definitely provide you the chance to lose a great percentage of tummy fat. Thus, this will help you lose weight in a very efficient way. Under this workout, you need to perform repetitions of dead lifts and you have to run for about 1.5 miles. This is being done in repetitions until you have already manifested some progress.

Dip is also among the best CrossFit exercises. This is a kind of exercise that will enhance the group of muscles in your body, not just one specific muscle. Like for example, ring dip routine will provide you additional balance and strength and at the same time, manage the stabilization of rings on the sides of your body. Therefore, expect that this will also immediately lose excess fat in your body.

If you are planning to undergo CrossFit training in the future, these are some of the exercises that you can perform. Every exercise mentioned will provide you great benefits. That is why it would be easy for you to achieve the body that you have always wanted to have. Once you experience the effects of the routines mentioned, you will surely tell yourself that this is way better than other programs from fitness institutions.

Chapter 5: 52 Insane Crossfit Workouts From Home And With No Equipment

These insane crossfit workouts are gathered from around the world and designed by experts and enthusiasts alike. Some you will like, others you will hate and a few will absolutely blow you away. Take take when performing these and as always stick to proper technique.3 Rounds for time: 10 Handstand push ups, 200 m run

Handstand 1 minute, hold bottom of the squat for 1 minute, 5 rounds.

6 Rounds for time: 10 push ups, 10 air squats and 10 sit ups

Run 1 mile, plus 50 squats-for time.

10 rounds for time: 10 push-ups, 10 squats, 10 sit ups

50 air squats, 4 rounds. rest for 2 minutes between rounds.

10 rounds for time: 10 push-ups, 100m dash

sprint 50 meters, 10 push ups. 10 rounds

5 rounds for time: 10 push-ups, 10 hollow rocks, run 200 meters

Handstand 10 seconds jack-knife to vertical jump. 25 reps...

10 rounds for time: 10 sit ups, 10 burpees

4 Rounds for time: 10 vertical jumps, 10 push ups, 10 sit ups

5 Rounds for time: 10 vertical jumps, run 400 meters

Sprint 200m and do 25 push ups, 3 rounds.

10 sets of 100 m dash (rest is length of time it took you to complete the last 100 m sprint)

100 air squats, rest 3 minutes, 100 air squats, rest 3 minutes, 100 air squats

5 Rounds: 30 second handstand against a wall, followed by a 30 second static hold at the bottom of the squat

"Susan" – 5 rounds for time: Run 200m, then 10 squats, 10 push ups

10 to 1 ladder: sit-ups/pushups and a 100 meter sprint between each set.

10 sets of: 30 second handstand hold followed by holding for 30 seconds at bottom of squat

10 x 50 meter sprint (rest is 2 minutes between sprints)

3 Rounds for time: 20 jumping jacks, 20 burpies, 20 air squats

4 Rounds for time: 20 ab mat sit-ups, 20 push-ups, 400 meter run

run 400m air squat 30 hand stand 30 seconds 3 rounds for time

3 Rounds for time: Run 1/2 mile, then 50 air squats

5 Rounds: 3 vertical jumps, 3 squats, 3 long jumps (rest as needed)

10 to 1 ladder: Burpees and Sit ups

10 Rounds for time: 10 burpees, 100 m sprint

For time: 100 jumping jacks, 75 air squats, 50 push ups, 25 burpies

5 rounds: 30 second handstand, 60 second squat hold (at the bottom of the squat)

3 x 20 tuck jumps, followed by 3 x 30 second handstand holds

3 rounds for time: 400m run/sprint followed by 30 air squats

4 sets x 25 jumping squats

3 rounds for form/technique: 5 handstand to jackknife to high jump, 5 handstand to jackknife to tuck jump, 5 handstand to jackknife to split jump

10 rounds for time: 10 walking lunges, 10 push-ups

3 Rounds: 30 push ups, 30 second handstand

Run 1 mile and at every 1 minute complete 10 air squats, 10 push-ups, 10 sit-ups

20 rounds: 5 push ups, 5 squats, 5 sit ups

10 Rounds: 5 push ups with a 30 second plebs plank (a hold at the top of the push up, arms extended and body tight like a plank!).

5 Rounds: 200 m dash (rest is the length of time it took you to complete the previous 200m dash)

50 air squats x 5. Rest equal amounts as it took to do each 50.

50 sit-ups, 400 meter run or sprint or walk. 3 rounds.

5 x 400M sprints (rest is the same time it took you to complete the last 400m sprint)

7 rounds for time: 7 squats, 7 burpies

Air squat x 10 push up x 10 sit up x 10 3 rounds for time

Air squatsx20, Burpiesx20, Push-Upsx20 – 3 rounds...for time bottom to bottom (rest at the bottom of the squat instead of standing....without support on your hands or butt and make the bottom good, straight back, butt back)

Do one air squat and take one breath, (you can breath all you want while you do the squat or squats) do 2 and take 2 breaths etc…up to 10, and then come back down to one.

Run 1 mile with 100 air squats at midpoint, for time

Handstand 5x 30 seconds. Run: 2x 800 meters for time. Do the handstands first. Rest and recover and do the runs with a rest in between that is as long as it took you to run your first 800.

Invisible Fran…21-15-9 of air squats and push ups for time.

Handstand to Jack-Knife to vertical jump. 30 Reps.

Run 1 mile and do 10 push-ups every 1 minute.

Run with high knees for 15 seconds and drop into a pushup, get back up and run with high knees again for 15 seconds…….repeat 5x. Each pushup counts as 1 rep. Rest. Do 3 more rounds.

Chapter 6: Getting Familiar With The Theory. The Basics.

Strength training is the repeated execution of the same movement at a relatively low pace (1 cycle in 1-5 seconds) and with significant external resistance. In this book, we employ the following terminology:

1) Locomotion - targeted control of body links with the help of muscles from the initial position to the final position and back to the original position.

2) Exercise - the sequential execution of several locomotions of the same type.

3) A series of exercises or a super series - a sequence of the same types of exercises or series with short (20-60 second) rest intervals.

4) Set - sequential execution of various exercises (series, super series) with short (1-3 min) rest intervals.

5) Superset - the sequential execution of a variety of exercises without a rest interval in

27

which the same muscles take part, with varying degrees of tension depending on the type of exercise.

Factors affecting muscle growth.

Practical studies have shown that when the working weight increases, the maximum possible number of projectile rises, or as they are also referred to, the repetition maximum, decreases. The weight with which you can perform only one repetition is taken as an indicator of the maximal strength of a given muscle group in a given exercise (in practice, this is also called a one-rep maximum). If the one-rep maximum is taken as 100%, then it is possible to construct a relationship between the weight of the projectile and the number of repetitions that an athlete can perform with this weight.

As I have already said above, the most important parameter of a muscle is the number of myofibrils in it, on which the strength and volume of muscle fibers depend. It can be said that the increase in strength is associated either with the development of the Central Nervous System (improvement of the processes of controlling the motor activity of the muscle), or with an increase in the number of myofibrils in the muscle that is under strain. An increase in their number leads to an increase in the cross-section of the muscle being worked out (the desired muscle mass growth).

Changes in muscle volume may also be associated with an increase in the mass of mitochondria, glycogen stores, and other cell organelles. It must be noted, however, that in a well-trained person, myofibrils and mitochondria occupy more than 90% of the muscle fiber, therefore the main factor of the the growth of the targeted muscle is an increase in precisely these components.

Considering everything said above, the goal of strength training is to increase the number of myofibrils in the muscle fibers. This process is possible with the acceleration of protein synthesis, even at the same old rate of its decomposition. Studies in recent years have revealed four main factors determining accelerated protein synthesis in the cell:

1) A reserve of amino acids in the cell.

2) An increased concentration of anabolic hormones in the blood (testosterone and the growth hormone, which are released in our body in response to serious psycho-physical stress).

3) An increased concentration of "free" creatine in muscle fibers.

4) An increased (just enough, but not excessive) concentration of hydrogen ions in the cell. This allows the hormones released during exercise to pass inside through the cell membrane.

The second, third and fourth factors are directly related to the content of the training exercises.

• The mechanism of synthesis of organelles in the cell, in particular of myofibrils, can be described as follows. During exercise, the ATP energy is wasted (in other words, the "mini power stations" of your body). The ATP energy expended by the body is replenished due to creatine phosphate reserves. There are two ways to replenish ATP energy, namely, glycolysis in the cytoplasm of the cell (muscle glycogen is mainly used to replenish ATP; the process takes place without the involvement of oxygen) and aerobic oxidation in the mitochondria (the process can take much longer, and oxygen is involved). Conventionally, all muscle fibers can be divided into two categories: Oxidative (those which contain a large number of mitochondria; the aerobic oxidation process predominates in these muscle fibers) and glycolytic (those which contain few mitochondria). In glycolytic muscle fibers, during anaerobic glycolysis, lactic acid is formed (a moderately high amount of it in the muscles causes an increase in the production of testosterone in the body and hypertrophy of the muscle itself; if excessively produced, it destroys the mitochondria of the cell, "acidifies" the body and has a harmful effect on the function of internal organs). Also, during this process, hydrogen ions accumulate in the cell (one of the main factors of muscle growth, which contributes to the penetration of anabolic hormones from the blood directly into the cell). The power of glycolysis is less than the costs of ATP, so the glycolytic muscle fiber gets tired rather quickly and loses the ability to go on with the exercise. Accordingly, if you want to have large and strong muscles, you can develop only glycolytic muscle fibers in the body, but if you want to get tough, strong muscles with a long endurance, you need to develop oxidative fibers.

Recent studies show that increasing the concentration of hydrogen ions causes an increase in the size of pores in the cell membranes, which leads to easier penetration of hormones into the cell (testosterone and the growth hormone, which increase muscle mass and bone density), activates the action of enzymes, and facilitates the access of hormones to hereditary information and DNA molecules. In response to a simultaneous increase in the concentration of creatine and hydrogen ions, informational RNA is formed more intensively (the structures formed on their basis are synthesized into cell organelles, in particular, myofibrils). Empirically, it has been established that myofibrils of the cell are synthesized best during long pauses (5 minutes or more) between strength approaches.

Theoretical analysis shows that when performing strength exercises until failure (for example, 10 squats with a barbell, one squat at a rate of 3-5 seconds, the exercise lasts up to 50 seconds), the following cyclic process occurs in the muscles: lowering and lifting with a barbell (1-2 sec) is performed at the expense of ATP reserves; in 2-3 second pauses, when the muscles become inactive (the load spreads along the spine and leg bones), ATP resynthesis from creatine phosphate reserves, and creatine phosphate is resynthesized due to the aerobic processes in oxidative muscle fibers and anaerobic glycolysis in glycolytic muscle fibers. Due to the fact that, as mentioned above, the power of aerobic and glycolytic processes is significantly lower than the ATP consumption rate in a given exercise, the creatine phosphate reserves are gradually exhausted, continuation of the exercise becomes impossible - a failure is reached. Simultaneously with the deployment of anaerobic glycolysis, lactic acid and hydrogen ions accumulate in the muscle. Hydrogen ions, as they accumulate, destroy bonds in the structures of protein molecules. This leads to a change in the activity of enzymes, an increase in the size of pores in membranes, and easier access of hormones to DNA. Excessive accumulation or an increase in the duration of the action of lactic acid even of not in very high concentrations, can lead to serious destruction, after which the destroyed parts of the cell will take a long time to be restored. Note, that an excessive increase in the concentration of hydrogen ions (which is distinctive of the so-called "glycolytic" or "killer" workouts with maximum acidification in a short period of time) leads to the destruction of the lysosome (a component of the cell containing various enzymes and acid). The enzymes secreted by the lysosome, in turn, contribute to the destruction of mitochondria and myofibrils in the muscle fiber. In particular, it was shown in the study of A. Salminen E.A. on rats, that excessively intense (glycolytic) running causes necrotic changes and a 4-5 fold increase in the activity of lysosomal enzymes. In other words, after such training your form deteriorates.

The combined action of hydrogen ions and free creatine leads to increased RNA synthesis. It is known that creatine is present in the muscle fiber during exercise and for 30–60 seconds after it, while creatine phosphate resynthesizes. Therefore, we can assume that for one set to the projectile, an athlete gains about one minute of pure time, during which informational ribonucleic acids are formed in his/her muscles. With the repetition of sets, the amount of accumulated informational ribonucleic acids will increase, but the concentration of hydrogen ions will increase simultaneously. In this regard, a situation may arise in which a greater number of organelles can be destroyed than later synthesized. This can be avoided by conducting approaches with large rest intervals (5 minutes or more) or if you train several times a day with a small number of sets in each workout. In this way, we can achieve a significantly greater stimulus for muscle growth than with standard training, while avoiding the negative effects of overtraining.

Recovery time.

The question of rest intervals between strength training days is related to the speed of realization of informational ribonucleic acids in cell organelles, in particular, in myofibrils. It is known that the informational ribonucleic acids themselves disintegrate in the first tens of minutes after the exercise, however, the structures formed on their basis are synthesized into organelles (myofibrils and mitochondria) within 4-10 days (depending on the amount of informational ribonucleic acid formed during training). In confirmation of this fact, one can recall the data on subjective sensations after a serious study of the muscle in an unfamiliar mode. The first 3-4 days there are violations in the structure of the myofibrils associated with strong muscle pains, then the muscle fiber normalizes and the pain disappears. Studies have also been conducted which showed that after strength training, the concentration of urea in the blood in the morning on an empty stomach is below the usual level for 3-4 days, which indicates the predominance of synthesis processes over degradation.

Breathing during exercises.

Studies by A.N. Vorobyov (1970-1980) showed that the implementation of exercises until muscle failure requires a special organization of breathing. The athlete shows the greatest strength when holding his breath and tensing, and he can demonstrate the least strength when exhaling, but, as you may know, it is very difficult to lift weights while inhaling. Therefore, in one locomotion we encounter the following sequence:

1) a short breath at the moment of holding the weight or lowering it (inferior to the functioning of the muscles);

2) holding the breath at the moment of contraction and while overcoming of the most difficult part of the trajectory;

3) exhale while reducing the load on the muscles.

Straining leads to an increase in intrathoracic pressure; the heart reduces in size up to 50%. This is caused both by the expulsion of blood from the cavities of the heart, and its insufficient inflow. At this moment, the heart rate rises from dormancy (70 beats) to 100 beats - this is without performing a power exercise, and the systolic (upper) pressure rises to 175-200 mmHg. The same high pressure is observed immediately after the power exercise and it relatively normalizes after a 1-3 minute rest period. Regularly performed power exercises produce reflexes that contribute to an increase in blood pressure before training while still at rest, and especially before competitions, and are, on average, MAP = 156, and DBP = 87 mm Hg. and for heavyweights, the pressure can be MAP = 170-180 mm Hg. Accordingly, if you have weak vessels, exercises with critical and near-critical weights is not advised.

Warning

It is obvious that strength exercises can be used in training only by absolutely healthy people, with arteries that don't show any signs of atherosclerosis. It is not difficult to imagine the situation when near-critical strength exercises are performed by a person with atherosclerotic plaques. An increase in pressure, an increase in the blood flow rate can lead to the separation of sclerotic plaques, their advancement along the vascular bed, blockage of arterioles. In this place a thrombus is formed, the tissues that are further along the channel stop receiving blood, oxygen and nutrients. This is when necrosis begins (the dying off of tissue). If this happens in the heart, then a heart attack occurs. A more serious condition, usually fatal, occurs when an arterial wall ruptures along with the detachment of the sclerotic skin.

Principles of sports training according to Seluyanov V.N.'s system.

Observance of the principles below will allow you to get the maximum results from practicing according to this objective: to achieve the ultimate improvements in your basic sports parameters (strength, speed, endurance, muscle mass), and to reach these achievements in the shortest possible way.

The principle of the choice and technique of exercises

Adherence to this principle requires a clear understanding of the biomechanics of the functioning of the musculoskeletal system in the chosen exercise. It should be understood that in some cases, non-observance of the exercise technique can lead to injury. For example, squatting with a heavy weight and your torso leaning forward may lead to injuries of the intervertebral discs of the lumbar spine.

The principle of quality effort

In each main exercise, it is necessary to achieve a maximum and full load. Adherence to this principle can be achieved when performing exercises in three versions.

1) The exercise is performed with an intensity of 90-100% of the one-rep maximum, the number of repetitions is 1-3. During this exercise and during the rest pause, there is no

significant accumulation of products that promote protein synthesis. Therefore, these exercises are considered as training of the neuromuscular control, the ability to manifest maximum effort in the chosen exercise. Exercises performed in this mode do not cause a noticeable increase in muscle mass.

2) In this mode, exercise is performed with an intensity of 70-90% of a one-rep maximum, the number of repetitions is 6-12 in one set. The duration of each exercise is 30-70 seconds. In this variant, the rule outlined above for the case of increasing the number of myofibrils in glycolytic muscle fibers is repeated, and it means that the exercise that is performed until muscle failure, which causes stress and the ultimate breakdown of creatine phosphate and. To increase this effect, you should follow various methods of intensifying the load at the end of the set. The greatest effect is achieved when performing the last 2-3 reps with the help of partners. Following this principle allows the athlete to achieve the maximum splitting of creatine phosphate so that free creatine and

hydrogen ions stimulate RNA synthesis, and the ultimate mental stress causes hormones to enter the blood from the pituitary gland and then from other glands of the endocrine system.

3) Performing "static-dynamic movements." The exercise is performed with an intensity of 30-70% of the one-rep maximum, the number of repetitions is 15-25 in one set. The duration of each exercise is 50-70 seconds. In this variant, each exercise is performed in a statodynamic mode. That is, without the complete relaxation of the muscles during the exercise. We work in partial amplitude and do not bring the muscles to the ending points. Tense muscles do not allow blood to pass through them, and this leads to hypoxia, lack of oxygen, and the unfolding of anaerobic glycolysis in active muscle fibers (within a specific muscle or muscle group). In this case, it is oxidative muscle fibers. After the first approach to the projectile, only slight local fatigue occurs. Therefore, after a short rest interval (20-60 s), the exercise should be

repeated. After the second approach, there is a burning sensation and pain in the muscle. After the third approach, these sensations become very strong - stressful. This leads to the release of large amounts of hormones in the blood, a significant accumulation of free creatine and hydrogen ions in the oxidative muscle fibers, which in turn, as we have said earlier, leads to hormones entering the cell and improving its functional component (synthesis of myofibrils and mitochondria).

The principle of negative movements

Muscles must be active in both contraction and lengthening, when performing negative work. That is, you need to strain the muscles as you overcome the load, and while accompanying the weight in the opposite direction.

The principle of unifying series.

This principle implies a system with a desire to reduce breaks (rest between sets) or the principle of the super series. For additional stimulation of the exercised muscles, a series of double, triple and multiple are used with little or no rest. The organization of exercises on the super series allows you to increase the residence time of free creatine in the oxidative muscle fibers, therefore more RNA should be formed in them. In this embodiment, the principle of pumping is also implemented - the essence of which is to increase blood flow to the muscle. According to Vader, this should lead to an influx of nutrients to the muscle, however, this point of view cannot be accepted. Filling the muscle with blood occurs in response to acidification (anaerobic glycolysis), hydrogen ions in the rest pause in such a muscle interact with hemoglobin and it releases carbon dioxide, which, in turn, affects the vascular chemoreceptors and leads to relaxation of the arteries and arterioles. Vessels expand and fill with blood. It does not bring any particular benefit, but this is a sure sign that the exercise was performed correctly, i.e. muscle fibers have accumulated a lot of hydrogen ions and free creatine, which ultimately will lead to an increase in muscle mass and athletic performance of the body.

Priority principle

In each workout, first of all, those muscle groups are trained, the growth of which hypertrophy is the goal. Obviously, at the beginning of the exercise, the hormonal background and endocrine system response are adequate, the stock of amino acids in the muscle fiber is maximum, therefore, the process of synthesis of RNA and protein proceeds at maximum speed.

Principle split or separate workouts

It requires the construction of a program (micro-cycle) of preparation in such a way that the developmental training for the same muscle group is performed 1-2 times a week. This is due to the fact that the construction of new myofibrils for 60-80% lasts 7-10 days. Therefore, supercompensation after strength training should be expected for 7-15 days. To implement this principle, the muscles are divided into groups. For example:

- Monday. Perform developmental training (4-9 approaches to the projectile), the extensor muscles of the back, trapezoid. The rest of the muscles are trained in a tonic mode (1-3 approaches to the projectile).

- Tuesday. Perform developmental training (4-9 approaches to the projectile), the extensor arm muscles, abdominal muscles are trained. The rest of the muscles are trained in a tonic mode (1-3 approaches to the projectile).

- Thursday. Perform developmental training (4-9 approaches to the projectile), the extensor muscles of the legs, the flexors of the arms. The rest of the muscles are trained in a tonic mode (1-3 approaches to the projectile).

- Friday. Perform developmental training (4-9 approaches to the projectile), flexor muscles of the joints of the legs are trained. The rest of the muscles are trained in a tonic mode (1-3 approaches to the projectile).

On each training day, certain muscle groups are trained.

Supercompensation system

Myofibrill mass growth requires 10-15 days. During this time, anabolic processes in the muscle fiber should unfold, and further continuation of the implementation of developmental training can interfere with the synthesis process. Therefore, to ensure the process of supercompensation, it is necessary to abandon the developmental exercises for 7-14 days and perform only tonic exercises, i.e. with 1-3 approaches to each projectile.

Principle of intuition

Chapter 7: Improving Training

on the system Seluyanov V.N.

Physiological analysis of strength exercises showed that they can be used only by absolutely healthy people. There is no doubt that the system of exercises from bodybuilding and other strength sports (as described above) is an excellent means of preventing the main types of human disease, since it stimulates the activity of the endocrine and immune systems (with the exception of overtraining). However, people with signs of atherosclerosis, diseases of the spine (osteochondrosis, radiculitis), thrombophlebitis, etc. cannot afford bodybuilding. For most people, it is necessary to develop a sparing system of strength exercises, which should keep everything positive in bodybuilding:

1) Stress causing an increase in the concentration of hormones in the blood;

2) Enhancement of anabolic processes in muscle tissue, formation of a muscular corset;

3) Increased catabolism in all tissues, and especially in adipose tissue, which leads to the renewal of organelles (which means ...), weight loss and treatment of the hereditary apparatus of cells.

The purpose of the system of health training according to Seluyanov V.N.

The goal is very simple - to make a person healthy, improve his health and performance, change body composition, that is, normalize the ratio of adipose and muscle tissue, increase the activity of men and women of a wide age range, improve immunity, and normalize the work of internal organs.

This system was developed on a scientific basis, that is, first, scientists studied how strength exercises affect the human body, then all Western training methods underwent a thorough analysis, including bodybuilding, aerobics, callanetics, and sports games. Were studied and Eastern health systems, such as yoga, qigong, martial arts. Some aspects were taken from the Russian physical therapy. In other words, all the most popular systems from the point of view of recovery of the organism have been subjected to research.

Further, using computer simulation, it was studied how and what kind of load favorably affects the human body, how the body's physiological systems respond to the load, what biochemical processes occur in the body when doing bodybuilding, aerobics, callanetics and other types of activities.

After the research, it became clear that none of these systems has a substantial theoretical basis. In addition, publications were discovered that experimentally proved the very low efficiency of the most popular systems of rehabilitation, such as different types of aerobics.

As a result, the VN Seluyanova health system was created or developed, which is based on the concept that the basis of human biological well-being (as a decisive health condition) is primarily the normal state of the endocrine and immune systems, as well as other physiological systems of the body. (cardiovascular, muscular, etc.), which, however, play a subordinate role in solving the problem of health.

The main principles of the improving system Seluyanov V.N.

The main means of physical education of the majority of practically healthy people, with the highest health-improving efficiency, are strength stat-dynamic, or isotonic exercises.

Regular use of static-dynamic exercises in a person's life creates conditions for increasing adaptive reserves, creates an increased and constant vitality.

Implementation of the ideas of recreational training on the system Seluyanova V.N. achieved with the following principles:

The principle of minimizing the growth of systolic blood pressure.

It is clear that for persons with signs of atherosclerosis it is contraindicated to perform exercises that cause an increase in blood pressure of more than 150 mm Hg. Therefore, when building a training session, you must observe the following requirements.

Warm up. Before the main part of the class, before strength exercises, it is necessary to achieve the expansion of the arteries and arterioles with the help of warm-ups. In this case, peripheral resistance is reduced, the work of the left ventricle of the heart is facilitated.

Exercise in the prone position. In the standing position, the heart must pressurize the blood in the arteries and arterioles to such an extent as to overcome the weight of the blood in the venous system, to raise the blood to the level of the heart. Therefore, we must give preference to exercises that are performed in the prone position.

Use the minimum amount of muscle in a power exercise. When performing dynamic exercises, straining and relaxing muscles facilitate the work of the heart. When performing strength exercises, when the pace is slow, the role of the muscular pump is reduced to a minimum, and with the activity of a large mass of muscles, with occlusion of blood vessels, the work of the heart becomes difficult. Therefore, in strength training, you should use the minimum number of muscles, especially if they work in a stat-dynamic mode.

Alternate exercises for relatively large mass of the muscles with the training of muscles with low mass. When building a set of exercises, it is often necessary to activate a large mass of muscles, which creates conditions for the growth of blood pressure. Therefore, the implementation of the following exercises for muscles with low mass eliminates possible problems with increasing blood pressure. For example, the execution of the block on the "triceps" after the bench press.

Perform stretching after each strength exercise or series. Stretching does not impose any particular difficulties on the cardiovascular system, therefore there are 10-40 seconds to reduce the activity of its activity. At the same time, muscle stretching stimulates the synthesis of protein in them.

How to do the exercises.

Exercises should be performed with constant muscle tension, without a relaxation phase, "to failure" or a burning sensation in the muscles. This is a signal to stop the exercise and rest. The amplitude of the movement is small. The exercise lasts 30-60 seconds, the rest between exercises for about 30 seconds. Here everyone fits individually, depending on their state. Exercises are performed at a moderate pace and without breathing.

For example, we do squats 10-20 times, rest 30 seconds, then repeat again 10-20 times. Again, rest 30 seconds, repeat the third time the same thing. Then rest on this muscle group for 5-10 minutes. At this time, you can work for example press, back or biceps in the same way. In one lesson, you can do 3-4 laps, and if you are well prepared, then 5-8 laps.

During one lesson, study 2-3 muscle groups no more. We are all different, so for each person should be their own individual approach. There are basic principles of training in the gym and they must be followed.

Another important point. Exercises should be performed so that there is no excessive acidification of the muscles (when the muscle hurts after leaving the hall). Hydrogen ions entering the muscle with strong acidification simply destroy the cell. Therefore, rest between exercises is important so that the lactic acid disappears and the synthesis of new cells begins.

The system of recreational gymnastics Seluyanova consists mainly of strength exercises, because the strongest hormone release into the blood occurs during strength exercises, when physiological stress is reached. Moreover, this is best done when performing the exercise in a static-dynamic mode.

What happens in the body when performing stat-dynamic exercises.

And that's what happens. When muscles are tensed, our body experiences short-term stress, and stress refers to everything that is unpleasant for our body, in this case - muscle tension.

In the cerebral cortex, mental stress arises, which excites the pituitary gland, and the pituitary gland is the endocrine system gland, which is located in the brain under the main cortex.

Other glands of the endocrine system begin to be activated. Glands of the endocrine system begin to secrete somatotropic hormone (or growth hormone), this hormone promotes the processes of synthesis in the body and activates protein, lipid, carbohydrate and mineral exchanges. This hormone builds the muscles, bones, ligaments and tendons of the body.

It is such an important hormone for men as testosterone. Women - estrogen. The main role of testosterone is to perform two important functions:

• Stimulate muscle growth, burn fat and maintain optimal bone density. Being anabolic steroid in its chemical structure, it activates the formation and renewal of cells and muscle structures

• Formation of a man of secondary sexual characteristics, ensuring the full activity of the organs of the reproductive system.

Estrogens in women are steroid hormones that affect the growth and development of the genital organs, preparing a woman for motherhood. If the female body contains estrogen in sufficient quantity, then the first thing that catches your eye is a beautiful figure with a thin waist and beautiful hips, velvety skin.

Here are two important hormones for us - growth hormone and testosterone (for women, estrogen), which the endocrine system begins to secrete during the exercise of static-dynamic exercises. Hormones enter the cell, and as described above, the construction of new cells and muscle structures begins, and fat deposits are burned. The body is updated. It is the endocrine system that is responsible for the healing of the body and plays an important role in human health.

Here is the subtitle!

•It should be noted that hormones do not enter into passive tissue, but into active (into that which is being worked out),

•Hormones appear only when there is mental stress or stress,

•If you engage with a barbell, then the weight should be 30-60% of the maximum weight that you can lift (from a one-repetitive maximum).

•Exercises should be performed without holding your breath.

•Between the exercises there should be a rest of 5-10 minutes so that the muscles recover and lactic acid leaves the muscles.

•The secreted hormones cleanse the blood vessels.

•Be sure to do a warm up before class 5-10 minutes and stretch

Theory of Atherosclerosis or "How to Clean the Vessels"

Using jogging will not get rid of atherosclerotic plaques, as there are no conditions for the release of hormones, no stress or mental stress. Jogging is an easy, comfortable jogging, without muscle tension.

Proper nutrition and regular release of hormones helps get rid of cholesterol plaques. The hormone penetrates the plaque, it lasts there for about a week, as a result, cholesterol is converted into fatty substances that go into the blood and are used for energy.

Performing physical exercises leads to activation of various tissues, strengthening of the processes of anabolism and catabolism in them. Depending on the diet, you can direct the course of adaptation processes in the desired direction, for example, increase muscle mass (intake is higher than the norm of complete protein), reduce the mass of adipose tissue (intake is below the norm of carbohydrates and fat).

Why not hold your breath during exercises.

When a person, when performing exercises, especially unprepared or aged, begins to hold his breath, he essentially deprives the heart of blood flow, the heart beats, and the blood does not flow properly.

After completing the exercise, the person gets up and begins to breathe intensively, the heart beats furiously, the pressure increases, the powerful blood flow hits the vessels, and if there is a cholesterol plaque there, then there is a chance that the blood flow will separate it from the vessel wall and block the smaller vessel. As a result, we get a microstroke. Therefore, holding the breath while performing static-dynamic exercises is unacceptable.

Selection of stat-dynamic exercises

When choosing stat-dynamic exercises, everyone needs to analyze their needs, goals, as well as limitations imposed by age or state of health. It is on the basis of these data that the training program will be compiled. For some, lighter exercises that are performed lying or sitting (for example, for people over fifty years old, in whom most of the muscles in the body do not have tone and strength) are suitable. Young people, full of strength and energy, may have a sense to take the exercises more difficult, use additional weight. The number of repetitions of exercises and approaches to the simulator (projectile) is also chosen individually. If the reader deems it necessary, then in the next book I will dwell on the exercises used in this system (although to put it briefly, any exercise from the gym can be used in a stat-dynamic mode), as well as on the number of repetitions and approaches for different groups (from age beginners to professional athletes).

Chapter 8: Bfr Training 101

The occlusion training bands should be applied right below the deltoid for the arms, or right below the hips on the quads. Also, they shouldn't feel terribly uncomfortable (a level 7 out of 10 in terms of tightness), and you shouldn't completely restrict all blood flow.

Most studies conducted on the value of occlusion training are similar to what you probably know as high-load training in terms of results. Studies show that, when compared to other types of training, occlusion-training results in greater development of muscle mass than without. BFR training also appears to increase muscle strength as well.

BFR Training Bands and How they work

So, how does it work? The premise is simple. When you workout using conventional methods, all of the metabolic byproducts of the workout move through and out of your body. With BFR training, the movement of the exertion hormones and by-products are restricted from leaving the limbs, forcing them to pool in or near the trained region. By doing this, several things occur in your body. First, your body will interpret this occlusion and, in an attempt to compensate, will release more of the anabolic growth hormones. The production of protein is also increased. Restricting blood flow during your workout also has been shown to aid in the repair of cells and tissues that are broken down during the workout cycle.

Second, by restricting blood flow to the muscles that you are focusing on, the smaller slow-twitch muscles fibers which rely on oxygen for energy starve out quickly, forcing the use and muscle damage of the fast twitch fibers – the fibers with the highest potential for growth. Type-II fast twitch muscle fibers are typically used during the final phase of a muscle contraction, not using oxygen, but by restricting blood flow the body must begin using the fast twitch fibers much sooner.

Occluded Blood Flow Technique

So, how should you train using this restrictive blood flow technique? Using your occlusion training bands, occlude the limbs of the area of the body you are focusing on. Tie it tight enough that it is mildly uncomfortable but not completely restricting all blood flow. This weightlifting technique is best used for a cycle of 4-8 weeks, or during the last week of each month as a de-load week to prevent overtraining.

BFR training is an extremely successful way to maximize your workout, allowing you to lift less weight and gain more muscle mass. It can be extremely painful and sometimes difficult, even when the load is light. It is an excellent way to grow and tone thigh, calf, and arm muscles. Studies have also shown that removing the occlusion during the workout to allow for a rush of the blood back to the muscle and the occluding it again does not produce a greater result, so it is better to leave the occlusion on during the entire workout.

The recommended load to lift during BFR is at least 30% (and no greater than 70%) of your maximum to achieve hypertrophy in the muscle and achieve the desired results. Considering several studies pertaining to this type of training, BFR training makes sense because major imbalances between muscle protein synthesis and muscle breakdown are the process that occurs during hypertrophy, the load lifted during the exercise is less important than what is actually occurring inside your body.

One other important key factor to consider is the release of various hormones as described previously. Several naturally occurring hormones are produced at an elevated rate during BFR. This elevation of hormone production has always been associated with acute resistance exercise routines with or without the restriction of blood flow, but the same product can be achieved with less work and to a higher degree.

BFR Training for Distant Muscle Groups

Muscle hypertrophy is what blood flow restricted studies have focused on. However, if you want to develop muscle groups apart from the occlusion sites like occlusion bands on upper arms, it may be good for you to use occlusion training.

This will be suitable if you want to increase your bench press strength and increase your chest muscle mass especially if you have an injury. Although it involves lighter weights, a new study has claimed that occlusion bench press helps to increase our muscle mass and strength if you have an injury or during inactivity.

Published in the Journal Clinical Physiology & Functional Imaging, the study examined the effect of restricting blood flow to the upper arm muscles especially during a low-intensity bench press workout. The study divided the volunteers into two groups.

One group was a control group while the other was a blood flow restricted group. For four weeks and six days every week, the two groups bench pressed 30 percent of their 1 repetition max (1RM) two times daily. There was a total of 75 repetitions during the workouts.

The group with the blood flow restricted bench pressed with elastic cuffs on both arms. It was noted that the pressure increase progressively on the two arms. External compression experienced an increase of 60 mmHg starting at 100 mmHg and ended at 160 mmHg.

The blood flow restricted group showed amazing results with an increase in muscle thickness experienced in the triceps, pectorals major ad an increase in the bench press strength. The triceps muscle thickness increased at a rate of 8 %, the pectorals major 16 % and the bench press increased to 6%. The control group 1RM bench decreased by 2%.

This study is applicable to individuals having an injury that affects their workout. The two groups in this study it should be noted were novices. With an injury, no advanced bench presser rains with 30% of his 1RM. When novices start their training, initial strength gains are neural. They get even better the movement pattern. Strength gain will take much longer because of the increased muscle mass.

Restricting blood flow to the upper arms while lifting light weights helps the bench presser to retain his or her muscle hypertrophy and also reach their maximum limit bench pressing strength.

Those people who are mostly travelling and cannot easily find heavy weights can also benefit from this. By incorporating occlusion training into your workout, you can use light weights and still gain muscle mass.

Frequently Asked Questions

Question: How tight exactly should the bands "feel" when I'm working out with them?

Answer: The bands should not actually feel as tight as you may think. The research suggests that you will attain the best results by tightening the bands to a level 5-7 on a scale of perceived tightness (10 being tightest). If the bands do not feel tight enough initially, you may need to increase your training volume (i.e. 30-50 repetitions, 3-10 sets) and decrease your rest intervals (i.e. 20-30 seconds rest). Also, since everyone's body type, shape, and density is unique, some may find our PRO bands or ELITE bands to be most suitable while others may find our CLASSIC model (which is more rigid) to be more suitable. See the last question for the key differences between each model.

Question: Is Occlusion Training safe?

Answer: Yes. There are numerous research studies to support that blood flow occlusion training is safe and effective. One study even states that occlusion training is safer than traditional weight training which is performed with heavier loads. Since occlusion training is performed with light weights only (~20% of 1RM), it puts significantly less stress on the nervous system (brain) and body. Also, you are already performing "occlusion training" whenever you are performing weight training since the occlusion is happening internally.

Question: Who is Occlusion Training best for?

Answer: Occlusion training can be especially useful for those looking to gain lean muscle mass without lifting heavy weights. This includes women who prefer not to lift heavy weights (at least not all the time), men who need a "deload" week for active recovery from traditional training (good to do at least one week every month), those recovering from injuries, and those just seeking rapid gains in muscle size. Also, since blood flow restriction training creates a bolus of blood and nutrients which flood the muscle/joint, it is theorized that it strengthens tissues (i.e.

ligaments and tendons). Stronger ligaments and tendons is great for injury prevention but also helps lower your brain's "threat" levels, which in turn makes your brain feel comfortable to increase your muscle strength contractile capabilities.

Question: How often should I perform Occlusion Training?

Answer: It is recommended to perform 4-5 days per week but for more rapid muscle hypertrophy gains it may be more effective to do every day, at least for the first 2-3 weeks. It is also something you can integrate into a current routine, such as on your rest days, as an active recovery week, or even at the end of every workout. The bands could even be worn every day on the legs while performing a light cardio routine for 30 minutes. With regard to aerobic activity, one study states "BFR aerobic (walking and cycling) exercise training methods have also recently emerged in an attempt to enhance cardiovascular endurance and functional task performance while incorporating minimal exercise intensity. Low-intensity BFR aerobic exercise [...] enhances muscle size and strength and simultaneously increases aerobic fitness."

Question: Where should I place the bands?

Answer: The BFR Bands can be placed on the upper arms (if training upper body) or upper legs if training lower body. Also, the bands to do not have to directly occlude an area to provide benefit.

For example, you will get the benefits of occlusion training for muscle groups like the chest and back when the bands are on the arms, even though they are not directly occluded.

Question: How many sets and repetitions should I be doing?

Answer: This all depends on the context of your goals, but generally you will see the best results performing 4-6 exercises for 3-10 sets each and 20-50 repetitions each. The weight used should of course be very light (only 20% of your 1 repetition maximum) and the rest period between sets should be short as well (20-30 seconds). Feel free to contact us anytime with questions.

Question: What are the main differences between the CLASSIC, ELITE, and PRO versions of the bands?

Answer:

CLASSIC Bands - just under 1 inch wide and made of a non-elastic material. These are great for a beginner to BFR training, and those with a body type that requires something more rigid.

ELITE Bands - 1.5 inches wide and made of a comfortable elastic material. These are great for the novice to BFR

training, and those with a body type that requires something more comfortable.

PRO Bands - 2 inches wide and made of an extra strong, durable elastic material. These are great for someone more advanced and those with more muscular body types. Because of the additional width, these can also work better the lower body.

Conclusion

SO – what do we take from all of this? Blood flow restriction can produce the same or better results with less work. Joints that are directly above the muscle groups that are the focus of the workout are tied off using occlusion bands allowing some blood flow. This type of exercise should only be augmentative, not a long-term replacement for traditional strength training, but you can "get more for less" by adding this as a supplemental workout to your regular routine.

Get after it,

P.S. If you're still not convinced, check out the research studies in the References section at the end of this book.

What you'll need:

PRO Bands - 2 inches wide and made

of an extra strong, durable elastic

material. These are great for someone

more advanced and those with more

muscular body types. Because of the

additional width, these can also work

better the lower body.

Buy them here:

=> bfrbands.com/order-pro/

ELITE Bands - 1.5 inches wide and made of a comfortable elastic material. These are great for the novice to BFR training, and those with a body type that requires something more comfortable.

Buy them here:

=> bfrbands.com/order-elite/

CLASSIC Bands - just under 1 inch wide and made of a non-elastic material. These are great for a beginner to BFR training, and those with a body type that requires something more rigid.

Buy them here:

=> bfrbands.com/order-classic/

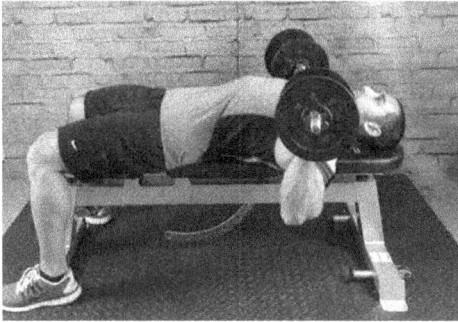

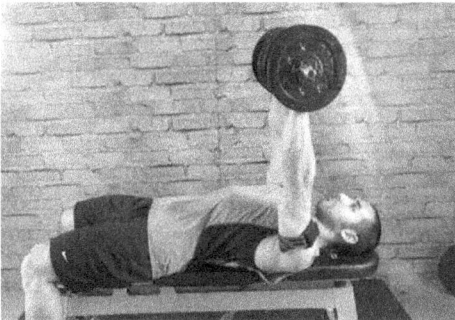

Biohacking Muscle

CHEST

With Blood Flow Restriction Training

1

DUMBBELL FLAT CHEST PRESS

Reps: 30,15,15,15

Sets: 2

Tempo: Slow / Moderate

Rest: 1 min

Notes:

Complete 30 reps, rest 30 seconds - 15 reps, rest 30 seconds - 15 reps, rest 30 seconds - 15 reps, rest 30 seconds. Loosen the bands and rest for 1 min, this is considered one set.

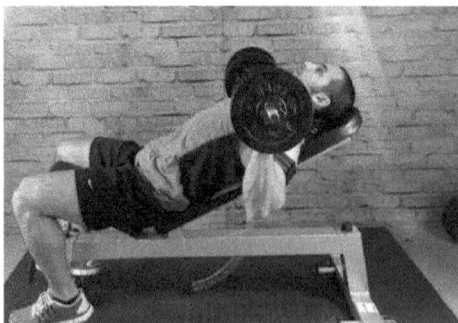

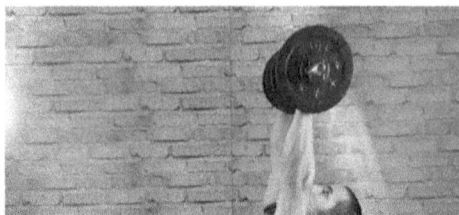

Biohacking Muscle

CHEST

With Blood Flow Restriction Training

2A

DUMBBELL INCLINE CHEST PRESS

Reps: 15, 15, 15

Sets: 2

Tempo: Slow

Rest: 1 min

Notes:

Complete 15 reps, rest 30 seconds - 15 reps, rest 30 seconds - 15 reps, rest 30 seconds - 1. Loosen the bands and rest for 1 min, this is considered one set.

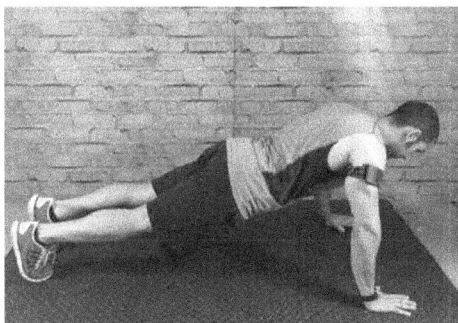

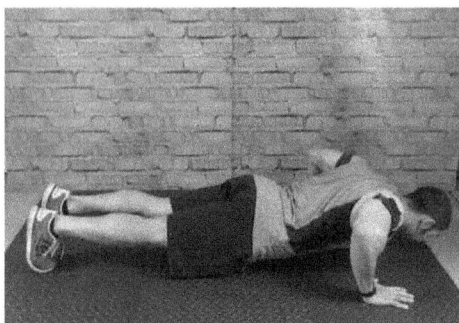

Biohacking Muscle

CHEST

With Blood Flow Restriction Training

2B

PUSH UPS

Reps: 25, 25, 25

Sets: 2

Tempo: Slow

Rest: 1 min

Notes:

Complete 25 reps, rest 30 seconds - 25 reps, rest 30 seconds - 25 reps, rest 30 seconds - 1.

Loosen the bands and rest for 1 min, this is considered one set.

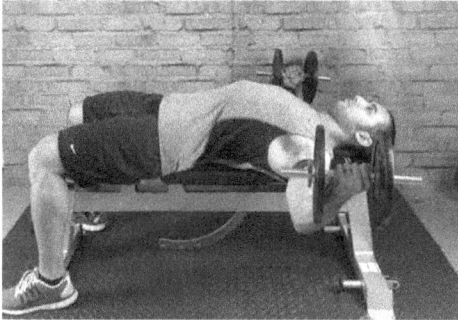

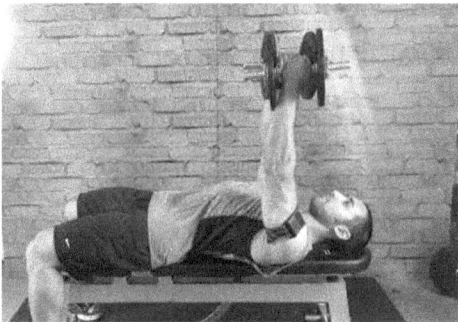

Biohacking Muscle

CHEST

With Blood Flow Restriction Training

3

FLYES

Reps: Drop sets - 20 (20% of 1RM), 25 (15% of 1RM), 30 (10% of 1RM) Sets: 3

Tempo: Moderate

Rest: none

Notes:

Perform these as drop sets, using 20% of 1RM (Rep Max) on the first set, then immediately to 25

reps with 15% of 1RM, and then immediately to 30 reps with 10% of 1RM.

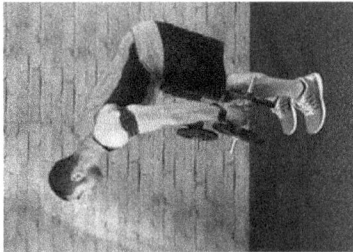

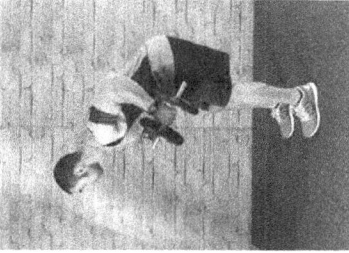

Biohacking Muscle

BACK

With Blood Flow Restriction Training

1

DUMBBELL BENT OVER ROW

Reps: 30,15,15,15

Sets: 2

Tempo: Slow / Moderate

Rest: 1 min

Notes:

Complete 30 reps, rest 30 seconds - 15 reps, rest 30 seconds - 15 reps, rest 30 seconds - 15 reps, rest 30 seconds. Loosen the bands and rest for 1 min, this is considered one set.

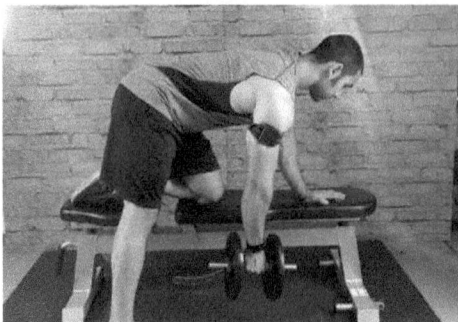

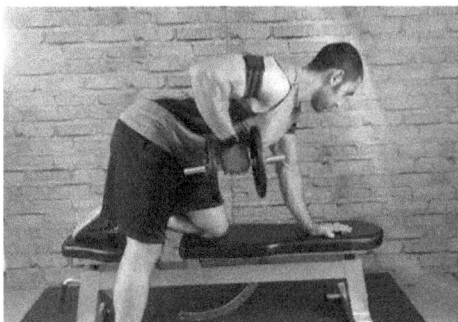

Biohacking Muscle

BACK

With Blood Flow Restriction Training

2A

ONE ARM ROW

Reps: 15, 15, 15

Sets: 2

Tempo: Slow

Rest: 1 min

Notes:

Complete 15 reps, rest 30 seconds - 15 reps, rest 30 seconds - 15 reps, rest 30 seconds - 1. Loosen the bands and rest for 1 min, this is considered one set.

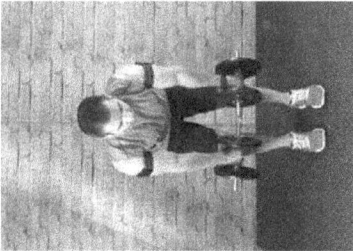

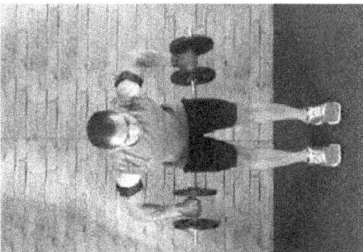

Biohacking Muscle

BACK

With Blood Flow Restriction Training

2B

BAND WIDE ROWS

Reps: 25, 25, 25

Sets: 2

Tempo: Slow

Rest: 1 min

Notes:

Complete 25 reps, rest 30 seconds - 25 reps, rest 30 seconds - 25 reps, rest 30 seconds - 1. Loosen the bands and rest for 1 min, this is considered one set.

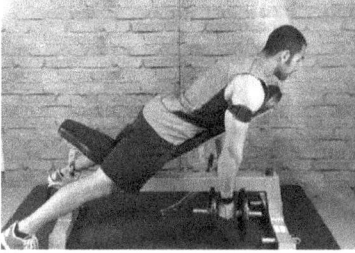

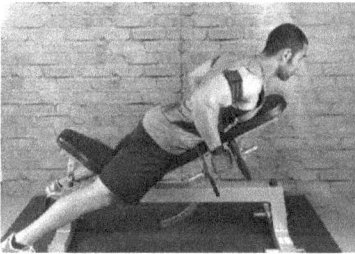

BACK

Biohacking Muscle

With Blood Flow Restriction Training

3

INCLINE BENCH ROW

Reps: Drop sets - 20 (20% of 1RM), 25 (15% of 1RM), 30 (10% of 1RM) Sets: 3

Tempo: Moderate

Rest: none

Notes:

Perform these as drop sets, using 20% of 1RM (Rep Max) on the first set, then immediately to 25

reps with 15% of 1RM, and then immediately to 30 reps with 10% of 1RM.

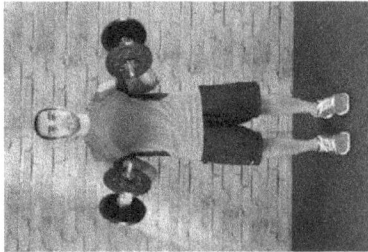

Biohacking Muscle

ARMS

With Blood Flow Restriction Training

1

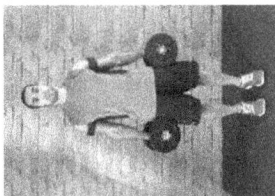

DUMBBELL CURLS

Reps: 30,15,15,15

Sets: 2

Tempo: Slow / Moderate

Rest: 1 min

Notes:

Complete 30 reps, rest 30 seconds - 15 reps, rest 30 seconds - 15 reps, rest 30 seconds - 15 reps, rest 30 seconds. Loosen the bands and rest for 1 min, this is considered one set.

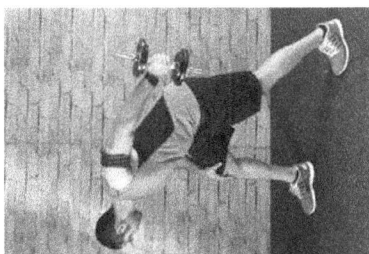

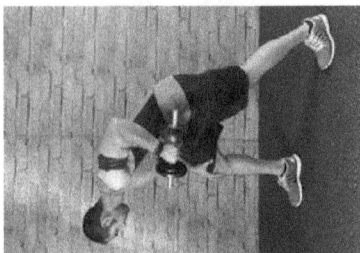

Biohacking Muscle

ARMS

With Blood Flow Restriction Training

2

DUMBBELL KICKBACKS

Reps: 30,15,15,15

Sets: 2

Tempo: Slow / Moderate

Rest: 1 min

Notes:

Complete 30 reps, rest 30 seconds - 15 reps, rest 30 seconds - 15 reps, rest 30 seconds - 15 reps, rest 30 seconds. Loosen the bands and rest for 1 min, this is considered one set.

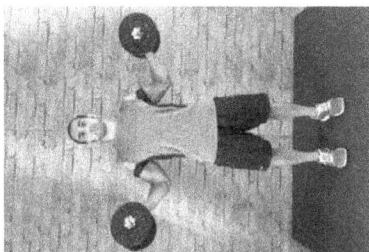

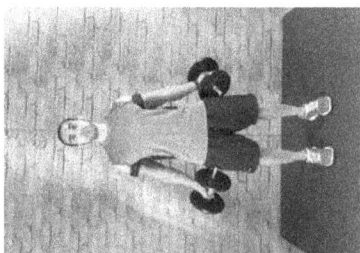

Biohacking Muscle

ARMS

With Blood Flow Restriction Training

3A

WIDE CURLS

Reps: 15,15,15

Sets: 2

Tempo: Slow

Rest: 1 min

Notes:

Complete 15 reps, rest 30 seconds - 15 reps, rest 30 seconds - 15 reps, rest 30 seconds - 1. Loosen the bands and rest for 1 min, this is considered one set.

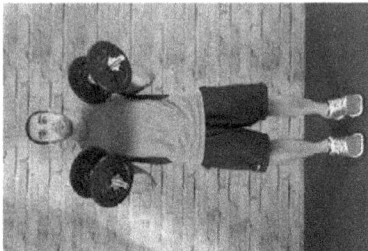

Biohacking Muscle

ARMS

With Blood Flow Restriction Training

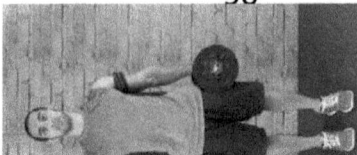

3B

HAMMER CURLS

Reps: 25, 25, 25

Sets: 2

Tempo: Slow

Rest: 1 min

Notes:

Complete 25 reps, rest 30 seconds - 25 reps, rest 30 seconds - 25 reps, rest 30 seconds - 1. Loosen the bands and rest for 1 min, this is considered one set.

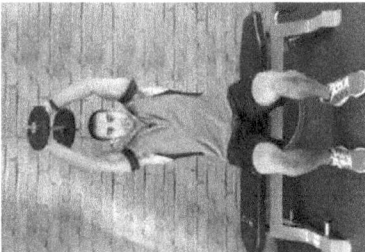

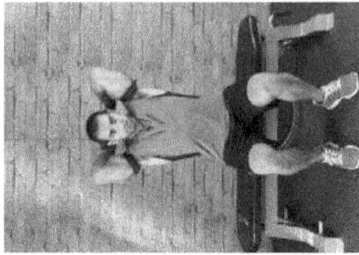

Biohacking Muscle

ARMS

With Blood Flow Restriction Training

4A

OVERHEAD DUMBBELL EXTENSION

Reps: 15,15,15

Sets: 2

Tempo: Slow

Rest: 1 min

Notes:

Complete 15 reps, rest 30 seconds - 15 reps, rest 30 seconds - 15 reps, rest 30 seconds - 1. Loosen the bands and rest for 1 min, this is considered one set.

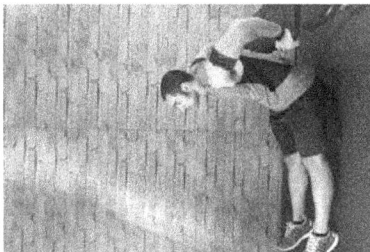

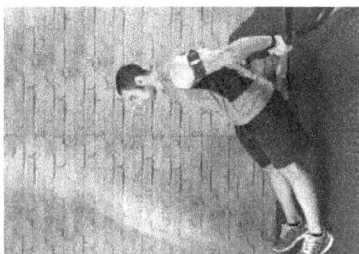

Biohacking Muscle

ARMS

With Blood Flow Restriction Training

4B

BENCH DIPS

Reps: 25, 25, 25

Sets: 2

Tempo: Slow

Rest: 1 min

Notes:

Complete 25 reps, rest 30 seconds - 25 reps, rest 30 seconds - 25 reps, rest 30 seconds - 1. Loosen the bands and rest for 1 min, this is considered one set.

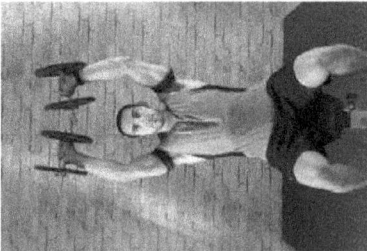

Biohacking Muscle

SHOULDERS

With Blood Flow Restriction Training

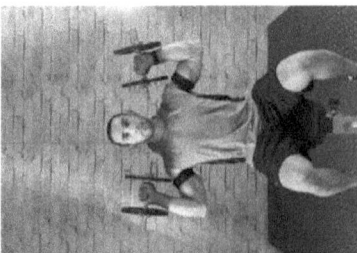

1

DUMBBELL SHOULDER PRESS

Reps: 30,15,15,15

Sets: 2

Tempo: Slow / Moderate

Rest: 1 min

Notes:

Complete 30 reps, rest 30 seconds - 15 reps, rest 30 seconds - 15 reps, rest 30 seconds - 15 reps, rest 30 seconds. Loosen the bands and rest for 1 min, this is considered one set.

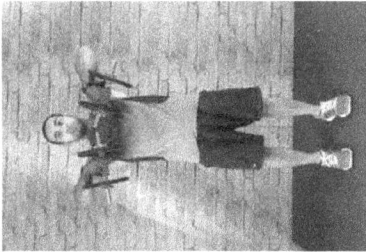

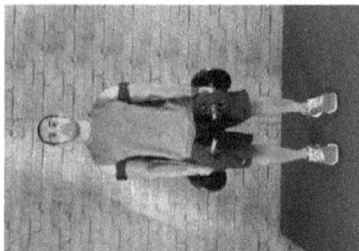

Biohacking Muscle

SHOULDERS

With Blood Flow Restriction Training

2A

UPRIGHT ROW

Reps: 15, 15, 15

Sets: 2

Tempo: Slow

Rest: 1 min

Notes:

Complete 15 reps, rest 30 seconds - 15 reps, rest 30 seconds - 15 reps, rest 30 seconds - 1. Loosen the bands and rest for 1 min, this is considered one set.

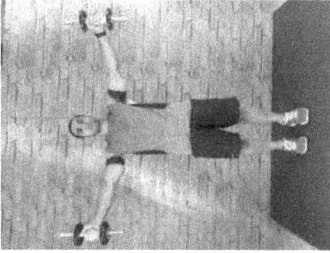

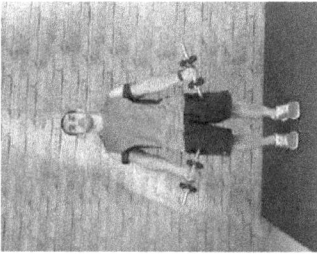

Biohacking Muscle

SHOULDERS

With Blood Flow Restriction Training

2B

DUMBBELL SCAPTION

Reps: 25, 25, 25

Sets: 2

Tempo: Slow

Rest: 1 min

Notes:

Complete 25 reps, rest 30 seconds - 25 reps, rest 30 seconds - 25 reps, rest 30 seconds - 1. Loosen the bands and rest for 1 min, this is considered one set.

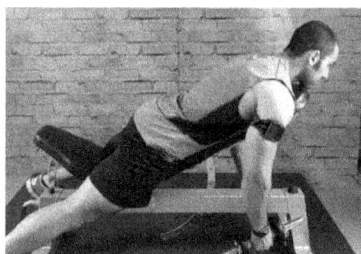

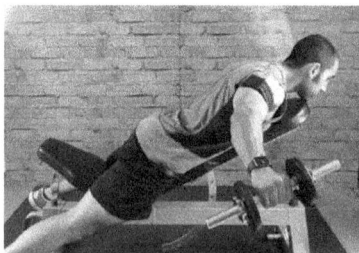

Biohacking Muscle

SHOULDERS

With Blood Flow Restriction Training

3

REAR DELT FLYES

Reps: 2Drop sets - 20 (20% of 1RM), 25 (15% of 1RM), 30 (10% of 1RM) Sets:

3

Tempo:

Moderate

Rest:

Notes:

Perform these as drop sets, using 20% of 1RM (Rep Max) on the first set, then immediately to 25

reps with 15% of 1RM, and then immediately to 30 reps with 10% of 1RM.

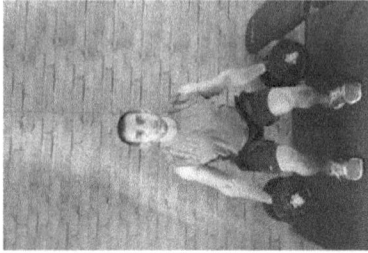

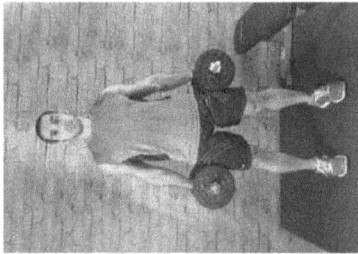

Biohacking Muscle

LEGS

With Blood Flow Restriction Training

1

DUMBBELL SQUAT

Reps: 30,15,15,15

Sets: 2

Tempo: Slow / Moderate

Rest: 1 min

Notes:

Complete 30 reps, rest 30 seconds - 15 reps, rest 30 seconds - 15 reps, rest 30 seconds - 15 reps, rest 30 seconds. Loosen the bands and rest for 1 min, this is considered one set.

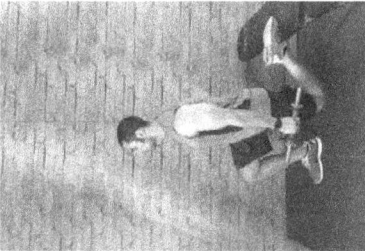

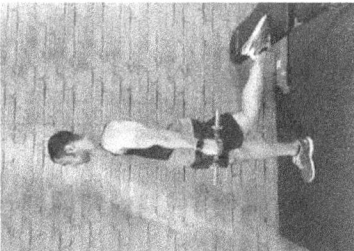

Biohacking Muscle

LEGS

With Blood Flow Restriction Training

2A

BULGARIAN SPLIT SQUAT

Reps: 15, 15, 15

Sets: 2

Tempo: Slow

Rest: 1 min

Notes:

Complete 15 reps, rest 30 seconds - 15 reps, rest 30 seconds - 15 reps, rest 30 seconds - 1. Loosen the bands and rest for 1 min, this is considered one set.

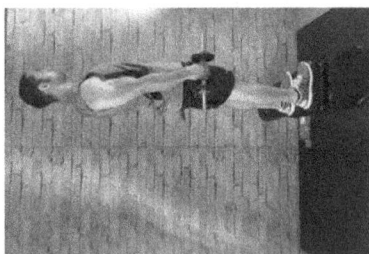

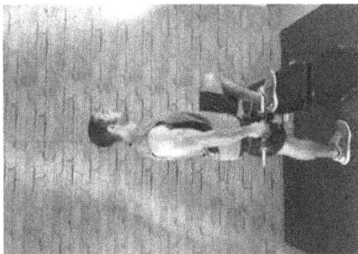

Biohacking Muscle

LEGS

With Blood Flow Restriction Training

2B

STEP UP TO BALANCE

Reps: 25, 25, 25

Sets: 2

Tempo: Slow

Rest: 1 min

Notes:

Complete 25 reps, rest 30 seconds - 25 reps, rest 30 seconds - 25 reps, rest 30 seconds - 1. Loosen the bands and rest for 1 min, this is considered one set.

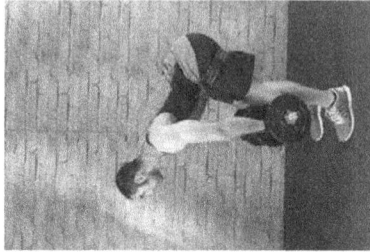

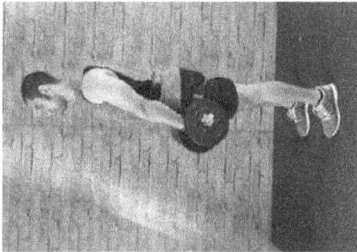

Biohacking Muscle

LEGS

With Blood Flow Restriction Training

3

STRAIGHT LEG DEADLIFT

Reps: Drop sets - 20 (20% of 1RM), 25 (15% of 1RM), 30 (10% of 1RM) Sets:

3

Tempo:

Moderate

Rest:

Notes:

Perform these as drop sets, using 20% of 1RM (Rep Max) on the first set, then immediately to 25

reps with 15% of 1RM, and then immediately to 30 reps with 10% of 1RM.

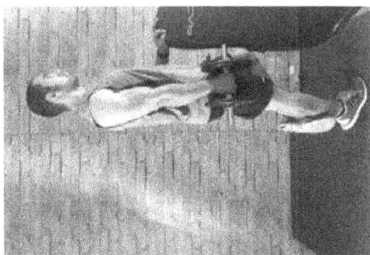

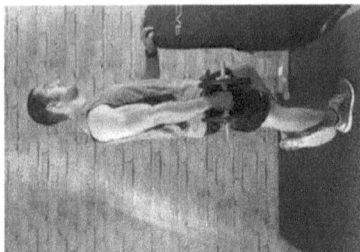

Biohacking Muscle

LEGS

With Blood Flow Restriction Training

4

CALF RAISE

Reps: 25,25,25

Sets: 2

Tempo: Slow

Rest: 1 min

Notes:

Complete 25 reps, rest 30 seconds - 25 reps, rest 30 seconds - 25 reps, rest 30 seconds - 1. Loosen the bands and rest for 1 min, this is considered one set.

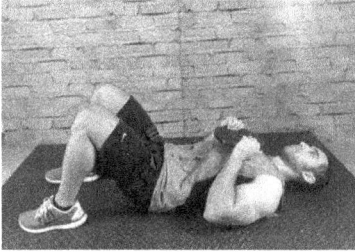

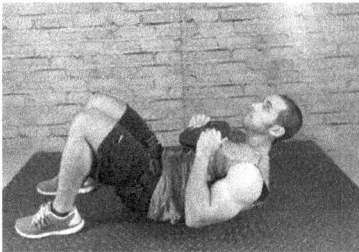

Biohacking Muscle

ABS

With Blood Flow Restriction Training

1

CRUNCHES

Reps: 30,15,15,15

Sets: 2

Tempo: Slow / Moderate

Rest: 1 min

Notes:

Complete 30 reps, rest 30 seconds - 15 reps, rest 30 seconds - 15 reps, rest 30 seconds - 15 reps, rest 30 seconds. Loosen the bands and rest for 1 min, this is considered one set.

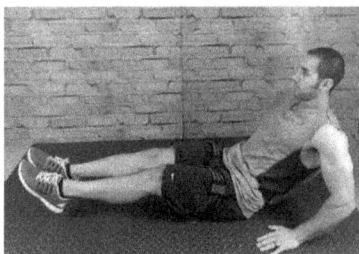

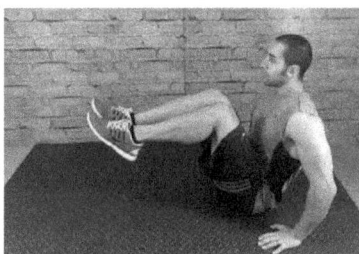

Biohacking Muscle

ABS

With Blood Flow Restriction Training

2A

REVERSE CRUNCH

Reps: 15, 15, 15

Sets: 2

Tempo: Slow

Rest: 1 min

Notes:

Complete 15 reps, rest 30 seconds - 15 reps, rest 30 seconds - 15 reps, rest 30 seconds - 1. Loosen the bands and rest for 1 min, this is considered one set.

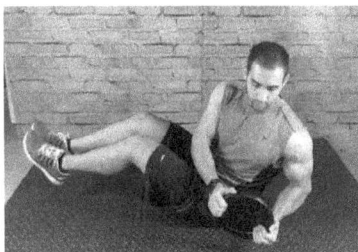

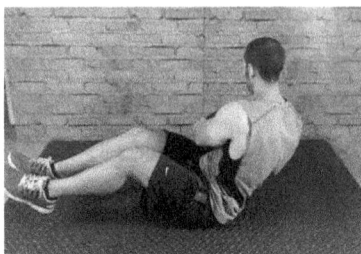

Biohacking Muscle

ABS

With Blood Flow Restriction Training

2B

RUSSIAN TWIST

Reps: 25, 25, 25

Sets: 2

Tempo: Slow

Rest: 1 min

Notes:

Complete 25 reps, rest 30 seconds - 25 reps, rest 30 seconds - 25 reps, rest 30 seconds - 1.

Loosen the bands and rest for 1 min, this is considered one set.

Frequently Asked Questions about BFR Training

Question: How tight exactly should the bands "feel" when I'm working out with them?

Answer: The bands should not actually feel as tight as you may think. The research suggests that you will attain the best results by tightening the bands to a level 57 on a scale of perceived tightness (10 being tightest). If the bands do not feel tight enough initially, you may need to increase your training volume (i.e. 3050 repetitions, 310 sets) and decrease your rest intervals (i.e. 2030 seconds rest). Also, since everyone's body type, shape, and density is unique, some may find our PRO bands or ELITE bands to be most suitable while others may find our CLASSIC model (which is more rigid) to be more suitable. See the last question for the key differences between each model.

Question: Is Occlusion Training safe?

Answer: Yes. There are numerous research studies to support that blood flow occlusion training is safe and effective. One study even states that occlusion training is safer than traditional weight training which is performed with heavier loads. Since occlusion training is performed with light weights only (~20% of 1RM), it puts significantly less stress on the nervous system (brain) and body. Also, you are already performing

"occlusion training" whenever you are performing weight training since the occlusion is happening internally.

Question: Who is Occlusion Training best for?

Answer: Occlusion training can be especially useful for those looking to gain lean muscle mass without lifting heavy weights. This includes women who prefer not to lift heavy weights (at least not all the time), men who need a "deload" week for active recovery from traditional training (good to do at least one week every month), those recovering from injuries, and those just seeking rapid gains in muscle size. Also, since blood flow restriction training creates a bolus of blood and nutrients which flood the muscle/joint, it is theorized that it strengthens tissues (i.e. ligaments and tendons).

Stronger ligaments and tendons is great for injury prevention but also helps lower your

brain's "threat" levels, which in turn makes your brain feel comfortable to increase your muscle strength contractile capabilities.

Question: How often should I perform Occlusion Training?

Answer: It is recommended to perform 45 days per week but for more rapid muscle hypertrophy gains it may be more effective to do every day, at least for the first 23

weeks. It is also something you can integrate into a current routine, such as on your rest days, as an active recovery week, or even at the end of every workout. The bands could even be worn every day on the legs while performing a light cardio routine for 30

minutes.

Question: Where should I place the bands?

Answer: The BFR Bands can be placed on the upper arms (if training upper body) or upper legs if training lower body. Also, the bands to do not have to directly occlude an area to provide benefit. For example, you will get the benefits of occlusion training for muscle groups like the chest and back when the bands are on the arms, even though they are not directly occluded.

Question: How many sets and repetitions should I be doing?

Answer: This all depends on the context of your goals, but generally you will see the best results performing 46 exercises for 310 sets each and 2050 repetitions each.

The weight used should of course be very light (only 20% of your 1 repetition maximum) and the rest period between sets should be short as well (2030 seconds). Feel free to contact us anytime with questions.

Question: What are the main differences between the CLASSIC, ELITE, and PRO

versions of the bands?

114

• CLASSIC Bands - just under 1 inch wide and made of a non-elastic material. These are great for a beginner to BFR training, and those with a body type that requires something more rigid.

• ELITE Bands - 1.5 inches wide and made of a comfortable elastic material. These are great for the novice to BFR training, and those with a body type that requires something more comfortable.

• PRO Bands - 2 inches wide and made of an extra strong, durable elastic material. These are great for someone more advanced and those with more muscular body types. Because of the additional width, these can also work better the lower body.

Important Disclaimer:

No express or implied warranty (whether of merchantability, fitness for a particular purpose, or otherwise) or other guaranty is made as to the accuracy or completeness of any of the information or content contained in any of the pages in this web site or otherwise provided by Exerscribe, Inc.

No responsibility is accepted and all responsibility is hereby disclaimed for any loss or damage suffered as a result of the use or misuse of any information or content or any reliance thereon. It is the responsibility of all users of this website to satisfy themselves as to the medical and physical condition of themselves and their clients in determining whether or not to use or adapt the information or content provided in each circumstance. Notwithstanding the medical or physical condition of each user, no responsibility or liability is accepted and all responsibility and liability is hereby disclaimed for any loss or damage suffered by any person as a result of the use or misuse of any of the information or content in this website, and any and all liability for incidental and consequential damages is hereby expressly excluded.

Chapter 9: Know What Crossfit Training Is

A hefty portion of games fans are getting to be keen on CrossFit preparing these days. Really, this preparation joins a great deal of powerful schedules that empower one to make differing qualities in workout. Then again, games medication specialists consider this preparation as an adjusted and comprehensive method for accomplishing wellness and wellbeing in simply a brief time of time. Like in picking up stamina, pick either to do swimming, biking and ball a few days in a week. In doing as such, an individual is permitted to appreciate a mixture of trainings which can be fun and energizing while getting the wanted wellness objectives.

Going back ever, CrossFit Training was begun by Greg Class, a secondary school tumbler who was alongside his wife named Lauren Glassman. CrossFit got to be connected with the first gym in 1995. In that same year, Santa Cruz police division employed Lauren Glassman to have the capacity to prepare the troops. For seven continuous weeks, the "Gagetown Infantry School" was concentrated in different tests in wellness classifications that incorporate quality, nimbleness, stamina, adaptability, parity, precision, velocity, force, coordination and respiratory perseverance. With the numerous classifications, CrossFit likewise scored the most noteworthy.

Thus, rec center mentors got to be fulfilled due to the workout results. Recreation centers that are subsidiary with CrossFit have become quickly. In 2005, there were just eighteen that rose to one thousand seven hundred recreation centers in 2010. Weightlifting mentors like Louie Simmons, Mike Burgener and Bill Starr joined forces with the CrossFit association.

Cross Fit is a wellbeing program that is incredibly intended to advance and convey the body to its top execution levels. In any case, the nature of this preparation system is not included with any of the dangers. As such, the advantages of CrossFit preparing far exceed the dangers. At the point when done in constrained time and in poor structure, diverse CrossFit activities may lift the danger of harm if performed erroneously. Along these lines, This ought not be performed by individuals without getting legitimate supervision first.

CrossFit And Its Effect On The Body- All of the parts of the human body are molded for them to capacity well. Through the activity varieties inside CrossFit preparing, the body is permitted to create different muscle bunches. The center is on a solitary gathering of muscles, as well as on all the body muscles also. Moving from a solitary movement to the following makes you practice the different muscles bunch for an adjusted preparing.

Crossfit activities might likely avert weariness. One of the basic issues in doing an activity regimen is the point at which you get to be exhausted. You all of a sudden get to be not keen on it that you ordinarily wind up stopping. Keep in mind that in CrossFit preparing, one can browse an extensive variety of activities every day, along these lines making the preparation all the more intriguing. With differed schedules, you can anticipate a mixture of workouts.

Crossfit preparing has no altered calendar, which makes it adaptable. On the off chance that circumstances have gone outside your ability to control, it might likely keep you from the customary morning runs in the city park. There are still gainful trainings that could be possible like swimming in the morning or playing yard tennis around evening time. The fortunate thing about it is that you can modify your preparation around anything you like.

So now that you have learnt somewhat about what CrossFit preparing is, now is the right time we secured the historical backdrop of this wellness wonder

Chapter 10: The Beginning Of Crossfit Training

Cross fit preparing is a type of physical preparing which is planned to add to your energy and your quality. This is a type of preparing which got to be famous in the year 2000. Due to the verifiable way of CrossFit activities, there are heaps of individuals who have been dependent on it. Indeed, this type of preparing is now picking up ubiquity nowadays. There are such a large number of individuals from the distinctive parts of the world why should energetic realize this preparation. Despite the fact that the general way of CrossFit preparing may be exceptionally sufficiently difficult, this routine merits performing. In the event that you are one of those individuals who are anticipating realizing this type of preparing, it is presently vital for you to know a tad bit of its history.

The real author of CrossFit preparing is Greg Glassman. He was an expert tumbler amid his time. In spite of the fact that the preparation has blasted in the year 2000, it began being offered by rec centers in the year 1995. The preparation itself concentrates regarding molding your body. This accompanies distinctive approachs which are planned to give general and expansive physical wellness through the heap of activities you can perform. Cases of the exercises under Greg Glassman are aerobatic, sprinting, weightlifting and others. These were essentially the first activities presented under this sort of activity. Be that as it may, new parts of the preparation have as of now been included. These have made the preparation more extraordinary and testing.

In particular, the first exercise center that has offered CrossFit preparing is CrossFit North, which is locafed in Seattle, Washington. The mentors who have contributed a ton in the improvement of CrossFit preparing are Mike Burgener, Bob Harpe and Louie Simmons. Notwithstanding that, there was an extraordinary assistance from Dr. Nicholas Romanov who is a topic master, that prompted the accomplishment of the preparation.

Romanov is the creator of Pose Method of running. In the late years, a few varieties have likewise been incorporated in the preparation. Among the people who are in charge of these progressions are Robb Wolf, Mark Rippetoe and Mark Twight.

Since the presentation of this type of preparing, such a large number of individuals have encountered real advantages of CrossFit preparing. Ordinarily, individuals who experience this type of preparing will experience improved adjusted, readiness, speed, adaptability, force and perseverance. Starting now, the ubiquity of this preparation is still at its tallness. In the year 2005, there were a sum of 15 exercise centers and wellness establishments offering this sort of preparing. In the compass of a half decade, the notoriety of the preparation even expanded. Based from the data discharged in the year 2010, there were 1,700 wellness foundations and rec centers offering this manifestation of preparing. It is likewise expected that the quantity of wellness organizations offering CrossFit preparing will keep on expanding nowadays. Starting now, it is normal that the quantities of wellness foundations and rec centers offering CrossFit preparing will expanded colossally for up to 3,400.

Path back in the year 1970, Greg Glassman did not have any sign that this preparation will be utilized following 3 decades. As indicated by one of his meetings, he principally added to this idea only for the purpose of his associates and obviously, himself. He never believed that some wellness lovers from alternate parts of the world will grasp the advantages of CrossFit preparing.

The greater part of those people who attempted this sort of preparing are very fulfilled by its outcomes in light of the fact that it drew out the best in them. Therefore, there are significantly more noteworthy quantities of health specialists who are mulling over the CrossFit preparing. Samples of these mentors who have committed some of their time in learning CrossFit preparing are Mike Burgener, Louie Simmons and Bill Starr who have prepared together with John Welbourn. When you complete this project, you will get affirmation classes concerning running and continuance, pot chimes, tumbling weightlifting and others. On the off chance that you need to realize this system, it is essential that you apply in a genuine teacher so you will be given the right preparing routines.

These are a portion of the things you have to remember concerning the historical backdrop of CrossFit preparing. Doubtlessly, it pays a ton to know a little foundation of this manifestation of preparing before you really do it. Dissimilar to alternate sorts of trainings, Greg Glassman never imagined that the world will admire this manifestation of activity than what he has envisioned. Through the years, expect that there will likewise be extra upgrades in this type of preparing. Without a doubt, these upgrades will improve CrossFit preparing a ton than in the recent past. Anyway, why not perform it now? You will doubtlessly attain to the body you have constantly longed for.

Chapter 11: How You Can Benefit From Crossfit Training

It is extremely great that there are more individuals who are getting to be wellbeing cognizant. Indeed, there are numerous men and ladies from everywhere throughout the world searching for the edge in the matter of wellness. So this is the place CrossFit preparing becomes an integral factor, Since this is an extremely powerful method for trim your body and increasing enormous wellness. So now we should find the advantages of CrossFit preparing

One of the advantages of CrossFit preparing is that it accompanies productive and quick results. Ordinarily, you just need to apply eventually in doing CrossFit preparing. Expect that toward the end of the preparation, you will recognize that your muscle has added to a more prominent quality and that your general wellness level has moved forward. You will likewise recognize that your energy has ended up better when contrasted with those individuals who make utilization of the customary workouts in wellness establishments. Then again, you need to verify that you perform the workout appropriately to experience its ideal impacts in simply a brief time of time.

Notwithstanding the rundown of advantages of CrossFit preparing, this is likewise a balanced sort of schedule. At the point when working out, it is essential to guarantee that your entire body is included. This is to guarantee that you have a proportioned and very much conditioned body not at all like the individuals who just concentrate in a particular piece of their body. Since CrossFit preparing makes utilization of an all encompassing methodology, expect that there are distinctive workout styles that will make your whole body fitter.

More often than not, wellness lovers have a tendency to trick and surrender in performing their schedules on the grounds that they feel exhausted with their schedule. On account of CrossFit activities, you won't feel exhausted. In each and every day, you can browse an assortment of workouts called WOD (Work Out of the Day). Indeed, you will never get exhausted and you may end up progressively getting to be occupied with your workouts step by step.

Another pleasant advantage of CrossFit preparing is that this is moderate. Regarding performing the activities you have to do, there is no requirement for you to secure distinctive hardware later on. The greater part of the parts of the workout get your body under way keeping in mind the end goal to accomplish a fitter build. This is far not the same as alternate sorts of schedules wherein you are obliged to buy your own particular gear for your activities to be performed effectively. Clearly, this is one of the advantages that you will like the most about this project.

Notwithstanding the advantages of CrossFit preparing said, this manifestation of preparing is likewise viable as far as molding your own particular body before experiencing any sort of schedule. This makes your body not able to feel

129

any anxiety. Before you are acquainted with another schedule, your coaches will first set up your framework through the presentation of some preparatory activity schedules. As you do the complex schedules later on, you won't encounter an excess of trouble. This is far diverse when contrasted with alternate sorts of activity schedules offered in some wellness foundations.

These are a portion of the advantages that you can get in performing CrossFit preparing. This is in reality a standout amongst the most encouraging schedules that you can attempt to issue you the sort of body you have for a long while been itching to have. It is vital that in the event that you need to experience the advantages of CrossFit preparing, you ought to just trust experience prepared specialists or teachers who will handle such preparing. This is a direct result of the way that the preparation is a particular type of activity. Without fitting abilities and learning about the system, it is unthinkable for you to experience the advantages of CrossFit preparing. Thus, now how about we turn to the distinctive activities of CrossFit!

Chapter 12: Crossfit Exercises

Cross fit preparing is considered as a progression of activities that is proposed to enhance your molding and quality. Fundamentally, CrossFit preparing concentrates principally in weightlifting under the Olympic style. There are distinctive schedules that you can do when you are wanting to attempt this manifestation of preparing. For the most part, the activities have the capacity to practice the majority of your body parts. As a result of the comprehensive methodology of this preparation, it would be simpler for you to accomplish the body that you have for the longest time been itching to have. On the off chance that you do experience this manifestation of preparing, it is essential for you to know a percentage of the CrossFit practices that you may do later on.

Cindy Routine is one of the CrossFit practices that can condition your body. Fundamentally, this is a type of full body activity and methodology, which incorporate pushups and additionally body weight squats. Cindy Routine accompanies a time allotment of around 20 minutes. This ought to be performed the following day, and the competitor ought to verify that advance is there. In spite of the fact that this routine can be performed rapidly, this is one of the best fat blazing schedules under CrossFit works out. Notwithstanding that, Cindy Routine is likewise planned keeping in mind the end goal to include additional mass of muscles in your midsection and in your shoulders. In this way, this issues you weight reduction and body designing impacts.

Messy 50 is additionally considered as one of the best CrossFit works out. Dissimilar to the first, this is an extremely requesting and thorough sort of workout. This obliges you to do 50 reiterations of 10 assortments of activities, for example, twofold unders, burpee, ball shots, back expansion, push press, lifts, rush steps, kettleball swings, draw ups and box hops. Regardless of the possibility that this sort of routine is profoundly requesting, it will at present offer your body with the speediest intends to get more fit and to blaze additional calories even in one session just. That is the reason weight reduction is doubtlessly one of the advantages of CrossFit preparing especially in performing this schedule.

Cross fit preparing is additionally made out of the activity called Thrusters and Pull Ups. This is additionally a workout that ought to be done in a dreary way. You can start the routine by executing the same number of push-ups and thrusters as you can. When you feel that you are as of now depleted and you have officially done all the most extreme reiterations, you can back off. This is an activity that is effective in smoldering the calories and abundance fats exhibit in your stomach zone.

L-sit is likewise included in the CrossFit practices that you can perform later on. In view of the way of this activity, it is best for your stomach and for your abs. For the most part, you can lose segment of your overabundance fat in stomach in performing this schedule. Under this work out, your body is being upheld by your arms while your legs are straight on your front.

Twofold Under is likewise another expansion to your CrossFit works out. This is essentially a type of hop rope practice that will expand the surge of your adrenaline. This is being performed by basically bouncing over the rope, guaranteeing that the rope will pass two times before you arrive on the floor. This routine will oblige you to have expanded work limit. Thusly, this will improve the calorie blazing impacts of the activity. Along these lines, this will issue you the opportunity to get in shape effectively.

Dead Lift Plus Run is likewise another segment of CrossFit preparing. The blend of running and dead lift makes this routine considered as an intense one. This will doubtlessly give you the opportunity to lose an incredible rate of tummy fat. In this manner, this will help you get more fit in an exceptionally productive manner. Under this workout, you have to perform reiterations of dead lifts and you need to run for around 1.5 miles. This is being done in reiterations until you have effectively showed some advancement.

Plunge is likewise among the best CrossFit works out. This is a sort of activity that will upgrade the gathering of muscles in your body, not only one particular muscle. Like for instance, ring plunge routine will give you extra adjust and quality and in the meantime, deal with the adjustment of rings on the sides of your body. Along these lines, expect that this will likewise instantly lose overabundance fat in your body.

In the event that you are wanting to experience CrossFit preparing later on, these are a percentage of the activities that you can perform. Each activity said will give you extraordinary advantages. That is the reason it would be simple for you to accomplish the body that you have for the longest time been itching to have. When you encounter the impacts of the schedules said, you will definitely let yourself know that this is path superior to different projects from wellness organizations.

Chapter 13: 52 Crazy Crossfit Workouts From Home And With No Equipment

These crazy crossfit workouts are accumulated from around the globe and outlined by specialists and fans alike. Some you will like, others you will loathe and a couple will completely clear you out. Take when performing these and as dependably stick to fitting strategy.

Workouts

3 Rounds for time: 10 Handstand push ups, 200 m run

Handstand 1 moment, hold base of the squat for 1 moment, 5 rounds.

6 Rounds for time: 10 push ups, 10 air squats and 10 sit ups

Run 1 mile, in addition to 50 squats-for time.

10 rounds for time: 10 push-ups, 10 squats, 10 sit ups

50 air squats, 4 rounds. rest for 2 minutes between rounds.

10 rounds for time: 10 push-ups, 100m dash

sprint 50 meters, 10 push ups. 10 rounds

5 rounds for time: 10 push-ups, 10 empty rocks, run 200 meters

Handstand 10 seconds pocketknife to vertical hop. 25 reps...

10 rounds for time: 10 sit ups, 10 burpees

4 Rounds for time: 10 vertical bounced, 10 push ups, 10 sit ups

5 Rounds for time: 10 vertical hops, run 400 meters

Sprint 200m and do 25 push ups, 3 rounds.

10 arrangements of 100 m dash (rest is period of time it took you to finish the last 100 m sprint)

100 air squats, rest 3 minutes, 100 air squats, rest 3 minutes, 100 air squats

5 Rounds: 30 second handstand against a divider, took after by a 30 second static hold at the base of the squat

"Susan" – 5 rounds for time: Run 200m, then 10 squats, 10 push ups

10 to 1 step: sit-ups/pushups and a 100 meter sprint between every set.

10 arrangements of: 30 second handstand hold took after by holding for 30 seconds at base of squat

10 x 50 meter sprint (rest is 2 minutes between sprints)

3 Rounds for time: 20 hopping jacks, 20 burpies, 20 air squats

4 Rounds for time: 20 abdominal muscle mat sit-ups, 20 push-ups, 400 meter run

run 400m air squat 30 hand stand 30 seconds 3 rounds for time

3 Rounds for time: Run 1/2 mile, then 50 air squats

5 Rounds: 3 vertical hops, 3 squats, 3 long bounced (rest as required)

10 to 1 step: Burpees and Sit ups

10 Rounds for time: 10 burpees, 100 m sprint

For time: 100 hopping jacks, 75 air squats, 50 push ups, 25 burpies

5 adjusts: 30 second handstand, 60 second squat hold (at the base of the squat)

3 x 20 tuck hops, took after by 3 x 30 second handstand holds

3 rounds for time: 400m run/sprint took after by 30 air squats

4 sets x 25 hopping squats

3 rounds for structure/procedure: 5 handstand to pocketknife to high hop, 5 handstand to folding blade to tuck hop, 5 handstand to folding blade to part bounce

10 rounds for time: 10 strolling lurches, 10 push-ups

3 Rounds: 30 push ups, 30 second handstand

Run 1 mile and at like clockwork finish 10 air squats, 10 push-ups, 10 sit-ups

20 adjusts: 5 push ups, 5 squats, 5 sit ups

10 Rounds: 5 push ups with a 30 second plebs board (a hold at the highest point of the push up, arms augmented and body tight like a board!).

5 Rounds: 200 m dash (rest is the period of time it took you to finish the past 200m dash)

50 air squats x 5. Rest equivalent sums as it took to do every 50.

50 sit-ups, 400 meter run or sprint or walk. 3 rounds.

5 x 400M sprints (rest is the same time it took you to finish the last 400m sprint)

7 rounds for time: 7 squats, 7 burpies

Air squat x 10 push up x 10 sit up x 10 3 rounds for time

Air squatsx20, Burpiesx20, Push-Upsx20 – 3 rounds… for time base to base (rest at the base of the squat as opposed to remaining… .without backing staring you in the face or butt and make the base great, straight back, butt back)

Do one air squat and take one breath, (you can breath all you need while you do the squat or squats) do 2 and take 2 breaths and so on... up to 10, and afterward return to one.

Run 1 mile with 100 air squats at midpoint, for time

Handstand 5x 30 seconds. Run: 2x 800 meters for time. Do the handstands first. Rest and recuperate and do the runs with a rest in the middle of that is the length of it took you to run your initial 800.

Imperceptible Fran... 21-15-9 of air squats and push ups for time.

Handstand to Jack-Knife to vertical bounce. 30 Reps.

Run 1 mile and do 10 push-ups at regular intervals.

Run with high knees for 15 seconds and drop into a pushup, get go down and run with high knees again for 15 seconds... ... .rehash 5x. Every pushup considers 1 rep. Rest. Do 3 more rounds.

Chapter 14: The Yearly Crossfit Games

As the CrossFit sensation has happened. It is just inexorable that contenders would need to ask the question...Who is the fittest? How would you know?

So Since 2007, the CrossFit Games have been made to answer these inquiries. Every year the occasion gets greater and greater as the against the best. Every last year the CrossFit amusements is a more complete test of wellness, and the competitors raise the level of rivalry to exceptional statures.

So in short the normal Games competitor in 2012 will be significantly more proficient than the world's best in 2007, as they've prepared the entire year round doing a wide range of diverse workouts to set up their psyche and body for whatever may come some way or another in the opposition.

A few extraordinary attributes characterize the CrossFit Games. As The Games change consistently, and the subtle elements are not reported until just before every occasion. Competitors will need to prepare year-round for a rival that is totally a secret.

Yet all is uncovered when they achieve the Home Depot Center, they put their preparation and mental mettle to the test and tackle a thorough, expansive running test of general physical limit. Following three days, the Fittest on Earth will have plainly separated themselves

The primary enormous news of the 2011 CrossFit Games season was the declaration that Reebok had consented to a 10 year sponsorship and on top of that they joined forces with ESPN to spread the game of wellness to a more extensive group of onlookers than any time in recent memory some time recently.

To start, ESPN3 secured the 2011 CrossFit Games with live three-hour shows running Friday, Saturday, and Sunday evenings.

After six weeks, ESPN2 ran 12 after generation shows covering the whole male and female rivalry on primetime TV. ESPN2 and ESPN re-circulated the demonstrates numerous times all through the fall and winter, fabricating new enthusiasm for the CrossFit Games as the group prepared for the 2012 Open

This new organization took into consideration an emotional increment in prize cash, from earlier years. The champs took home a joined $1 million prize satchel, with the male and female individual victors taking home $250,000 each.

The 2011 Reebok CrossFit Games season started with the first ever Open rivalry. Competitors overall contended in six workouts as the weeks progressed, posting their scores continuously and on the web. Anybody could toss their cap in the ring to vie for a position among the fittest competitors on the planet. More than 26,000 competitors contended in the Open, making it one of the biggest donning occasions ever.

game is brought into more nations and more individuals need to test their wellness levels

Chapter 15: Getting Started.

As with most endeavors in life, fitness is achieved through smart, tiered progression. it is never expect a child to do well in algebra without having mastered basic arithmetic. Likewise the best CrossFit boxes would never expect you to put a barbell of any significant weight above your head without having mastered the skill of properly picking up a 10 pound medicine ball of the ground." – Scott Pfeifer

If you are new to CrossFit, the best way to develop this base of strength and coordination is to start with learning the following foundational CrossFit movements.

• Running

• Kettlebell swing

• Ring row

• Pull up

• Push up

- Rowing

- Air squat

- Shoulder press

- Deadlift

- Clean

- Front squat

- Snatch

The aims, prescription, methodology, implementation, and adaptations of CrossFit are collectively and individually unique, defining of CrossFit, and instrumental in our program's successes in diverse applications.

Aims

From the beginning, the aim of CrossFit has been to forge a broad, general, and inclusive fitness. Looking at all sport and physical tasks collectively, what physical skills and adaptations would most universally lend themselves to performance advantage. Capacity culled from the intersection of all sports demands would quite logically lend itself well to all sport.

Prescription

The CrossFit prescription is "constantly varied, high-intensity, functional movement." Functional movements are universal motor recruitment patterns; they are performed in a wave of contraction from core to extremity; and they are compound movements—i.e., they are multi-joint. They are natural, effective, and efficient locomotors of body and external objects. But no aspect of functional movements is more important than their capacity to move large loads over long distances, and to do so quickly. Collectively, these three attributes (load, distance, and speed) uniquely qualify functional movements for the production of high power. Intensity is defined exactly as power, and intensity is the independent variable most commonly associated with maximizing favorable adaptation to exercise. Recognizing that the breadth and depth of a program's stimulus will determine the breadth and depth of the adaptation it elicits, our prescription of functionality and intensity is constantly varied. We believe that preparation for random physical challenges—i.e., unknown and unknowable events—is at odds with fixed, predictable, and routine regimens.

There are three main energy systems that fuel all human activity. Almost all changes that occur in the body due to exercise are related to the demands placed on these energy systems. Furthermore, the efficacy of any given fitness regimen may largely be tied to its ability to elicit an adequate stimulus for change within these three energy systems. Energy is derived aerobically when oxygen is utilized to metabolize substrates derived from food and liberates energy. An activity is termed aerobic when the majority of energy needed is derived aerobically. These activities are usually greater than ninety seconds in duration and involve low to moderate power output or intensity. Examples of aerobic activity include running on the treadmill for twenty minutes, swimming a mile, and watching TV.

 Energy is derived anaerobically when energy is liberated from substrates in the absence of oxygen. Activities are considered anaerobic when the majority of the energy needed is derived anaerobically. These activities are of less than two minutes in duration and involve moderate to high power output or intensity. There are two such anaerobic systems, the phosphagen system and the lactic acid system. Examples of anaerobic activity include running a 100-meter sprint, squatting, and doing pull-ups

It warrants mention that in any activity all three energy systems are utilized though one may dominate. The interplay of these systems can be complex, yet a simple examination of the characteristics of aerobic vs. anaerobic training can prove useful. Aerobic training benefits cardiovascular function and decreases body fat. This is certainly of significant benefit. Aerobic conditioning allows us to engage in moderate/ low power output for extended period of time. This is valuable for many sports.

Athletes engaging in excessive aerobic training witness decreases in muscle mass, strength, speed, and power. It is not uncommon to find marathoners with a vertical leap of several inches and a bench press well below average for most athletes. Aerobic activity has a pronounced tendency to decrease anaerobic capacity. This does not bode well for athletes or the individual interested in total conditioning or optimal health. Anaerobic activity also benefits cardiovascular function and decreases body fat. Anaerobic activity is unique in its capacity to dramatically improve power, speed, strength, and muscle mass. Anaerobic conditioning allows us to exert tremendous forces over a very brief time. Perhaps the aspect of anaerobic conditioning that bears greatest consideration is that anaerobic conditioning will not adversely affect aerobic capacity! In fact, properly structured, anaerobic activity can be used to develop a very high level of aerobic fitness without the muscle wasting consistent with high volume aerobic exercise.

Before you commit, ask yourself some questions including:

What are your fitness goals? Would CrossFit be the right fit to reach those goals?

Do you do well training in group environments? (Some people prefer to workout solo or with a partner.)

Will you actually go to classes regularly? After all, those classes will be expensive if you frequently blow them off.

Do you do better with one-on-one training? You might be better with a personal trainer if sharing an instructor among many participants limits you.

Are you fully committed to your time at CrossFit? (You might prefer the go-at-your-own-pace at a regular gym.)

Does the potential cheerleading attitude at CrossFit motivate you? (If high-fiving someone makes you roll your eyes, you might come across as aloof or unfriendly during workouts.)

These are also questions to bring up when you talk to your instructor. CrossFit isn't for everyone, and you've got plenty of other workout options to reach you goals.

Chapter 16: Benefits Of Crossfit Training.

No new fitness program has had quite the impact of CrossFit. Chances are you've heard about it, and all the stuff that goes with it. You'll have heard strange vocabulary like 'Boxes' (CrossFit gyms), 'WODs' ('workouts of the day') and much more. You might have friends or colleagues that have taken up CrossFit and even tried new diets or fitness challenges through their 'Box'. It might sound kind of intimidating, or you might think it's just another fitness fad, but CrossFit has a lot going for it and is definitely here to stay.

Benefit #1: It's Convenient

When starting on a fitness journey, many people struggle with whether to join a gym, invest in a home fitness studio, or hire a personal trainer. CrossFit gives you some of the benefits of all three of these.

CrossFit Boxes will provide you with all of the equipment you need for a variety of all-around workouts. Cardio equipment, free weights, flexibility aids - all of these are at your CrossFit Box. Unlike a public gym though, you don't have to figure them out on your own. Your CrossFit classes will be well guided by trained coaches, with skills support, someone to check your form and prevent injuries, and pre-planned workouts so you don't have to think about your own program. Because CrossFit Boxes typically serve small groups that train regularly, you get a much more tailored program than if you try an online fitness program or work out on your own at the gym. Best of all, the group structure means you get most of the attention of a personal trainer, but at a fraction of the price.

If you have been thinking about training at home because you like the convenience and the privacy, CrossFit might work for you too. Most Boxes run very small groups, so you won't be working out in front of a lot of people. Typical groups are around six people, and chances are you'll find everyone in your group is supportive and encouraging. Most Boxes offer classes and groups from early hours until late in the evening, so you'll find a time and days that work for you. CrossFit Boxes are now a global phenomenon, so there's bound to be one near you, and you can usually find Boxes to visit when you are traveling too!

Benefit #2: You'll Get Strong

One of the cornerstones of CrossFit is strength training. Not every workout is lifting weights but expect to get familiar with free weights and weight lifting techniques. Don't think CrossFit is all about 'bulking up' - it's much more subtle than that, and it isn't going to give you huge biceps.

The CrossFit strength training exercise is primarily designed to help you get toned and get strong. Of course, that will help you to look good, and if weight loss is part of your goals then improving muscle tone will certainly help you too. CrossFit strength training uses a varied, all-around program based on a few basic movements, so don't worry about having to learn lots of new skills. You'll soon master the basics of 'Olympic lifting' technique, and chances are you'll be surprised at how much fun weightlifting can be, and how quickly you see the benefits!

CrossFit is about all-around 'functional fitness.' The strength training you'll do at the Box will not only get you stronger and fitter, it will help prevent injury in other sports and activities. Best of all, you'll enjoy that newfound strength in your everyday life, whether it's picking up your toddler, moving the sofa, or just impressing your friends!

Benefit #3: You'll Get Fit

CrossFit isn't just about lifting weights. Most workouts follow the premise of the 'High Intensity Interval Training' (HIIT) model, where you work out - hard - for short periods interspersed with rest. Sure, you'll have 'strength days' where your WOD (workout) is primarily about lifting heavy and lifting correctly, but on other days your WOD will be totally different. These high intensity days will introduce you to a cardio workout that is much tougher, and more fun, than just running on a treadmill or joining a spin class. Best of all, you'll get a serious workout in a much shorter time.

CrossFit prides itself on combining the cardio benefits of HIIT with strength training for maximum benefits. While you can expect to run from time to time, run distances are short (a half mile or less) and interspersed with other intensive movements based on plyometrics and explosive power. Your cardio WODs might have you pulling tires, carrying sandbags, jumping onto boxes, and throwing weighted balls. If you've shied away from cardio workouts because you didn't think you could do them, but you still want to get fit, then CrossFit is perfect. Some workouts push you very hard, but in short intervals that really anyone can do (called 'Tabata' workouts), and over time you'll find that your speed, power, and endurance all improve!

Benefit #4: You'll Get Flexible

Okay, let's say you are looking at the schedule for your local CrossFit Box, and you see most classes are about an hour. We've just been describing the types of high intensity workouts you can expect, and you may be thinking, 'I need to work that hard for an hour?' Well, no. Remember how we said with powerlifting and with HIIT workouts you get a lot of benefit from a shorter workout time? You'll work out hard for about half an hour, but your class will start and finish with a very carefully designed program of warm up and cool down that protects your muscles and joints and helps prevent injury.

These aren't your everyday stretching routines though, CrossFit warm ups and cool downs do much more. Based on the premise that to prevent injury and maximize performance you need to build a combination of flexibility (muscle movement) and mobility (joint range and stability). This means that what you get is so much more than just improved flexibility, you get another aspect to your workout that helps you stay active for longer!

Benefit #5: It's Fun

One of the best things about CrossFit workouts is the variety. This is not the kind of program where you turn up and do pretty much the same workout over and over, or just run on a treadmill. Like we've mentioned, workouts are designed to build into a complex progression of strength, cardio, and flexibility training, but most of all they focus on 'functional fitness'. That means CrossFit WODs can sometimes be really creative.

Benefit #6: CrossFit is Lifestyle Coaching

CrossFit is more than just a workout program; it really is a way of life. Some Boxes include yoga or Pilates sessions, meditation programs, and personal enrichment plans. These programs are designed to work with the fitness elements of CrossFit. You don't have to become a true 'CrossFitter', but if you are looking for an all-around, whole body and mind improvement package, CrossFit might be perfect for you. Because it's a lifestyle program, CrossFit encourages a community approach to help you stay motivated and achieve your goals. CrossFit athletes are encouraged to support each other, and your fellow Cross Fitters will pick you up after a tough workout and help you celebrate after a WOD personal best. Don't be surprised if your CrossFit coach also takes a personal interest in your success. They may call you if you miss a workout to make sure you're okay and they'll let you know if they see anything changing - positively or negatively - in your progress. Not only will you enjoy the camaraderie of your local Box, you'll get access to an entire online community that shares your interests!

Benefit #7: You Can Even Compete

Not everyone works out to train for an event, but there's no doubt that a certain amount of competition can help you stay motivated and enthusiastic about your workouts. The great thing about CrossFit is you can be as competitive - or not - as you like.

How to Start Doing CrossFit Workouts

If you choose to visit a CrossFit center or follow a protocol you find online, you'll find that CrossFit workouts are usually done by following the "Workout of the Day," also called the WOD. WODs can seem a bit confusing if you're new to CrossFit, so here's how they work:

First, it helps to get the basic terminology down. A "rep" (or repetition) is one iteration of a movement, such as one bench press or one squat. A "set" is a group of reps, such as 10 reps or squats. Each WOD usually features a certain number of sets of various movements. The pattern is to complete the sets, rest, repeat, rest, repeat and so on.

The amount of time for resting between sets depends on a few different factors, like your ability to recover and the primary goal of the WOD. Sometimes you might want to try having your WOD be timed, so in this case your rest time between sets would likely be shorter so you can complete the entire CrossFit workout quicker. If you attend a class at a CrossFit Box, a WOD description might be written in several different ways. For example, doing a WOD in

161

"rounds" would translate to doing a set of several exercises, resting and then repeating the whole circuit again. As an example, this type of WOD could be written as "21-15-9" which would indicate you perform one exercise 21 times, followed by another exercise 21 times and so on. Then you start from the beginning and do the first exercise 15 times, second exercise 15 times, etc.

If you choose to do a CrossFit-style workout on your own, start by practicing moves you're more familiar with without added weights. Begin gradually by doing lower reps, until you become more physically able to handle higher reps or adding additional weight.

Chapter 17: Nutrition For Crossfit Training.

For several decades now, bad science and bad politics have joined hands to produce what is arguably the costliest error in the history of science—the low-fat diet. This fad diet has cost millions unnecessary death and suffering from heart disease, diabetes and, it increasingly seems, a host of cancers and other chronic and debilitating illnesses. A new age is dawning in nutrition: one where the culprit is no longer seen as dietary fat but excess consumption of carbohydrate—particularly refined or processed carbohydrate. In fact, there's an increasing awareness that excess carbohydrates play a dominant role in chronic diseases like obesity, coronary heart disease, many cancers, and diabetes. This understanding comes directly from current medical research. Amazingly, the near universal perception that dietary fat is the major culprit in obesity has no scientific foundation.

Additionally, excess consumption of carbohydrate may soon be shown to be linked to Alzheimer's, aging, cancers and other disease through a process known as "glycosylation". At any rate, a search on "Google" for "hyperinsulinemia" reveals hundreds of ills linked to this metabolic derangement. The rapidly growing awareness of the consequences of elevated blood sugar is one of the more promising avenues of medical advancement today. Though frightening, the diseases brought about through hyperinsulinemia can easily be avoided by minimizing carbohydrate consumption—specifically carbohydrate that gives substantial rise to blood sugar and consequently insulin levels. There is a singular measure of carbohydrate that gives exactly this information—"Glycemic Index." Glycemic index is simply a measure of a food's propensity to raise blood sugar. Avoid high glycemic foods and you'll avoid many, if not most, of the ills associated with diet.

In the Zone scheme, all of humanity calculates to either 2-, 3-, 4-, or 5-block meals at breakfast, lunch, and dinner, with either 1- or 2-block snacks between lunch and dinner and again between dinner and bedtime. We've simplified the process for determining which of the four meal sizesand two snack sizes best suits your needs. Being a "4-blocker", for instance, means that you eat three meals each day where each meal is composed of 4 blocks of protein, 4 blocks of carbohydrate, and 4 blocks of fat. Whether you are a "smallish" medium-sized guy or a "largish" medium-sized guy would determine whether you'll need snacks of one or two blocks twice a day.

Once you determine that you need, say, 4-block meals, it is simple to use the block chart and select four times something from the protein list, four times something from the carbohydrate list, and four times something from the fat list every meal. One-block snacks are chosen from the block chart at face value for a single snack of protein, carbohydrates, and fat, whereas two block snacks are, naturally, chosen composed of twice something from the carbohydrates list combined with twice something from the protein list, and twice something from the fats. Every meal, every snack, must contain equivalent blocks of protein, carbohydrate, and fat. If the protein source is specifically labeled "non-fat", then double the usual fat blocks for that meal.

To determine your block, follow the chart below

Chapter 18: Crossfit Training Workouts.

BEGINNER WORKOUTS

However, for many, initially starting can be a daunting process. But it shouldn't be. What's more, once you start getting the hang of it, you won't be able to stop and you'll wonder why you didn't start sooner. The combination of high-intensity circuits, staple CrossFit moves and some good old-fashioned weight training will keep your muscles continually guessing. Don't rest between moves but recover for one minute after each cycle. Repeat five times. For the uninitiated, Crossfit is a strength and conditioning programme that involves constantly varied, functional movements – lifting, climbing, rowing, sprinting, and more – done at high intensity. To pump up the burn, you also use equipment such as barbells, gymnastic rings, kettlebells and medicine balls.

1.Barbell deadlift

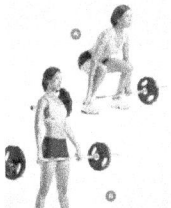

Sets: 5

Reps: 10

Rest: None

Squat down and grasp a barbell with your hands roughly shoulder-width apart. Keep your chest up, pull your shoulders back and look straight ahead as you lift the bar. Focus on taking the weight back onto your heels and keep the bar as close as possible to your body at all times. Lift to thigh level, pause, then return under control to the start position.

2.Barbell squat

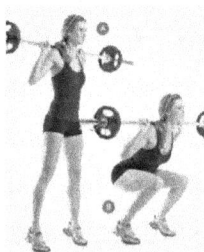

Sets: 5

Reps: 10

Rest: None

Stand with your feet more than shoulder-width apart and hold a barbell across your upper back with an overhand grip – avoid resting it on your neck. Hug the bar into your traps to engage your upper back muscles. Slowly sit back into a squat with head up, back straight and backside out. Lower until your hips are aligned with your knees, with your legs at 90 degrees – a deeper squat will be more beneficial but get the strength and flexibility first. Drive your heels into the floor to push yourself explosively back up. Keep form until you're stood up straight: that's one.

3. Kettlebell swings

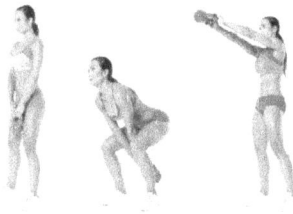

Sets: 5

Reps: 30 secs

Rest: None

Place a kettlebell a couple of feet in front of you. Stand with your feet slightly wider than shoulder-width apart and bend your knees to lean forward and grab the handle with both hands. With your back flat, engage your lats to pull the weight between your legs (be careful with how deep you swing) then drive your hips forward and explosively pull the kettlebell up to shoulder height with your arms straight in front of you. Return to the start position and repeat without pauses.

4. SUMO DEADLIFT HIGH PULL-UPS

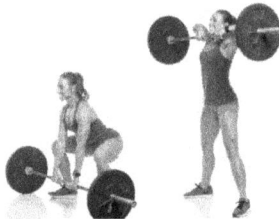

Sets: 3

Reps: 10

Rest: None

Stand with feet shoulder-width apart. Hold centre of bar with hands shoulder-width apart. Push hips back and lower into deep squat. As you do so, slowly lower bar until it reaches mid-shin. Keep bar close to body at all times. Jump and shrug shoulders with straight arms to lift bar to chest level. Bring elbows to ear level, pointed towards ceiling. Slowly lower bar and return to starting position.

Tip: Do the jump-and-shrug This quick action transfers power from hips to trapezius. By lifting bar by a few centimetres, bringing it just underneath the chin becomes easier.

5. AIR SQUAT

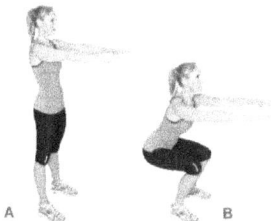

A   B

Start doing air squats properly and not only will bulletproof your body, you'll get more out of your squat.

Step 1: Stand with your feet hip-width apart with your toes pointed slightly outward. Your arms should be hanging loose by your side. Then engage your core muscles and push out your chest slightly by pulling your shoulder blades towards each other.

Step 2: Bend your knees and squat down as if you were sitting into a chair. Keep your weight on your heels and keep your core tight. Your eventual goal will be to touch your glutes to the back of your calves but if you can only get to parallel right now, that's fine. Make an effort to keep your knees externally rotated (don't let them collapse inward). As you lower down, you can either raise your arms straight in front of you or keep them bent in front of your chest. Focus on keeping your torso upright and core tight.

Step 3: Straighten your legs and squeeze your butt to come back up, lowering your arms back to your side.

6. FRONT SQUAT

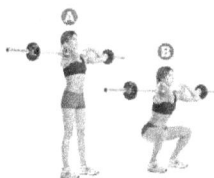

Step 1

Set up under the bar by grasping it with a closed overhand grip slightly wider than shoulder-width. Place bar evenly on top of your front deltoids and collarbone.

Step 2

Remove your thumb and pinky finger from under the bar and keep a relaxed, open palm, with 3 fingers under the bar.

Step 3

Remove the bar from the rack and take a step or two backward. Take a breath in and hold that breath towards the bottom to maintain intra-abdominal tightness. Flex hips and knees slowly. Remember to drive your knees outwards as you squat down also.

Step 4

As you reach the bottom, be sure to continue to squeeze the elbows up and inwards. Focus on keeping your elbows up at the bottom of the lift.

Step 5

Once you've reached parallel, drive upwards but keep heels on floor and knees aligned with feet. Halfway up, let your breath out, and power through with the glutes and core braced to the top position. Tip: Use a loose grip Rest bar on your fingertips if you can. This lets you offload the weight from wrists to body.

7.DEADLIFT

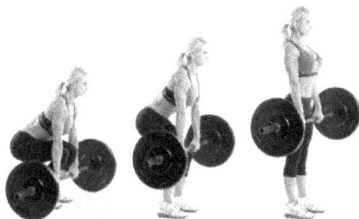

Stand with feet hip-width apart. Hold bar with hands placed wider than shoulder-width apart.

Push hips back and lower into deep squat. As you do so, slowly lower bar until it reaches mid-shin. Keep bar in contact with body at all times. To return to standing position, do the same steps in reverse.

7. BENCH PRESS

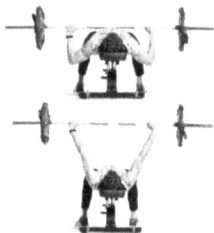

The bench press has always been an important exercise for bodybuilders, strength athletes and powerlifters. It is an effective movement for introducing pressing strength to beginners.

BENEFITS

Hard active work for the chest, shoulders and arms, isometric work for the forearms

A very good place to learn how to bear weight and support a weighted movement

Especially useful for building upper body and tricep strength

TECHNIQUE

Shoulders back on the setup/rear delts resting on the bench

Bring the weight over the chest (not above the eyes)

Shoulders tight on the setup leading to a tight arch in the back

Break the bar on the way down: puts elbows in the right position

Spread the bar with the hands on the way up: activates the triceps

Wide feet/pushing feet into the ground/ spreading the floor with the feet

Don't have a bench? Execute this movement while lying on the floor. The floor press, often called the "poor man's bench," will still increase your pressing power.

8. PULL UP

The pull-up is considered a true measure of strength by many trainers and with good reason. Completing a correct pull-up uses all the muscles of the back and arms and is a very effective upper body exercise.

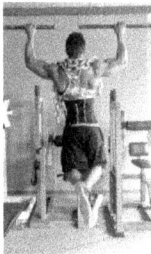

BENEFITS:

177

pullups are one of the most convenient exercises. You can do them everywhere.

pullups do a great job of targeting the back and biceps

it engages the back, shoulders, chest and arms.

helps developing powerful forearms and grip strength to help improve your performance in several sports

TECHNIQUE STEP-BY-STEP:

Step 1: Grab The Bar. Grip it about shoulder-width apart. Full grip with your palms down.

Step 2: Hang. Raise your feet off the floor by bending your knees. Hang with straight arms.

Step 3: Pull. Pull yourself up by pulling your elbows down to the floor. Keep your elbows close.

Step 4: Pass The bar. Pull yourself all the way up until your chin passes the bar. Don't do half reps.

Step 5: Repeat. Lower yourself all the way down until your arms are straight. Breathe. Pullup again.

INTERMEDIATE WORKOUTS

Am I Ready for Intermediate CrossFit?

You are ready for intermediate CrossFit workouts if:

You have been consistently practicing CrossFit for at least four months

You perform the workout three to five days a week

You can identify the nine fundamental movements, which include the Squat, Front Squat, Overhead Squat, Press,Push Press, Push Jerk, Deadlift, Sumo Deadlift High Pull,and Medicine Ball Clean

The intermediate level CrossFitters are at a pivotal point in their training. They have most of the movements down and can perform a majority of the workouts as prescribed without having to scale exercises or weights; however, they are lacking in strength or ability in a number of areas which is stunting their overall progress as an athlete. They are unable to reach to that next level because of these deficiencies and so they feel they are no longer improving.

For these athletes, creating a realistic but challenging indicator list will be critical. Setting new PRs or failing to PR will prove where the athlete has been focusing his/her attention and where they need to spend more time.

Here is a list of exercises for the Intermediate level CrossFitter to monitor:

1. C2B pull-ups

2. Handstand push-ups

3. Rope climbs

4. Ring dips

5. Squat cleans

The Kettlebell Swing

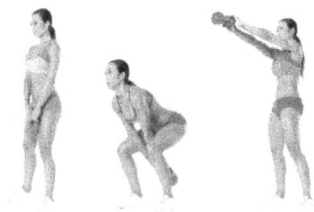

Once you have mastered the basic squat, sometimes referred to as the air squat, you are ready to add power and agility with the kettlebell swing. This ball-shaped cast iron weight, is one of the most favored strength training tool within the fitness industry. As a highly maneuverable CrossFit accessory, it provides a challenging, albeit efficient and effective way to train the arms, shoulders, back and lower body.

Why You Need It

The kettlebell swing increases the intensity of the squat and arm thrust movements, by increasing work load and repetitions. While it appears to rely on momentum, don't be deceived. Absolute precision is required, in order to avoid thrusting the kettlebell into over-extension.

The Full Snatch

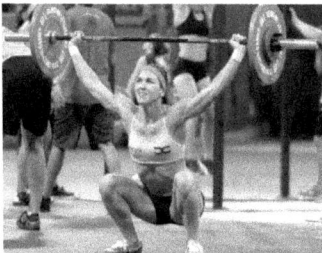

Everything you learned in the CrossFit basics was preparing you for the full snatch exercise. The snatch is an Olympic power lifting move. It requires you to begin in a low squat position, then lift a weighted straight bar over your head. All of the major muscles in your body are called into action during the full snatch.

Why You Need It

As its highly descriptive name implies, you have to snatch the bar and lift it over your head as you simultaneously extend your legs into a standing position The full snatch demands skill, concentration, coordination and flexibility along with accurate timing for injury prevention. These skills easily transfer to daily life and athletic activities. If your aspirations include one day competing in the CrossFit games, mastery of the full snatch is imperative.

Before You Begin

Many of the CrossFit intermediate exercises feature gymnastic-type movements, including handstands, combined with push-ups or explosive plyometric jump mixed in with squats and short-distance sprinting. For safety reasons, initiate your CrossFit program with the help of a fully trained professional in the method. If your trainer does not offer alignment or muscle imbalance feedback, seek help elsewhere.

ADVANCED WORKOUT

These Crossfit workouts will help you to test and improve your strength and build muscle. Real strength and muscle is built gradually over time in line with intelligent programming, but it's always a good idea to keep your body guessing and stress it in new ways.

1. CrossFit Total

"Wanna find out how strong you are? You need to test your one rep max to see where you stand right now," Salveo says. The CrossFit Total is the sum of the highest load lifted of three fundamental moves: the back squat, shoulder press, and deadlift.

To work up to your one-rep max, you'll warm up and then take three attempts, with plenty of rest between. For the first attempt, choose a heavy weight you know you can do for three reps. For the second attempt, choose a load you know you can do for a single rep based on the load of the first attempt. For the final lift, attempt the weight you want to do based on your performance on the previous two attempts.